Clinical Pharmacology:
The Essential Principles Made
Simple and Useful

Samuel Matthews

Clinical Pharmacology: The Essential Principles Made Simple and Useful, First Edition

ISBN 978-0615964973

CONTENTS

Preface

Pharmacology is a vast topic. Although there are literally thousands of different drugs, the drugs in each class generally work the same way, have the same side-effects and contraindications, among other similarities. This book provides a general overview of pharmacology.

Samuel Matthews

CHAPTER 1

INTRODUCTION TO PHARMACOLOGY

Pharmacology is not conceptually difficult. Many drugs can be divided into two main categories: 1) those that mimic or enhance normal biological processes, and 2) those that block or antagonize normal biological processes. Drugs that mimic or enhance biological processes include adrenalin, insulin, and albuterol. Drugs that block or antagonize biological processes include some high blood pressure medications such as some alpha blockers, beta blockers, and diuretics; some antipsychotics, anesthetics, and most antiarrhythmia drugs.

Of course drugs have more formal divisions than "those that mimic or enhance..." and "those that block or antagonize...." Yet, this generality can be helpful in understanding how most drugs work. For example, the sympathetic nervous system tries to maintain adequate blood pressure when a person is in shock by releasing adrenalin. Generally speaking, the drug dobutamine mimics adrenalin to maintain adequate blood pressure and cardiac output.

As a separate example, the parasympathetic system naturally slows a person's heart rate. During bradycardia, (abnormally slow heart rate) blocking the parasympathetic system's influence on the heart allows the heart to beat faster. Atropine blocks or antagonizes the parasympathetic nervous system's influence on the heart, thus increasing heart rate because the sympathetic system, which normally increases heart rate, is left unopposed to increase the heart rate.

Most biological processes (blood pressure, blood sugar, arthritis) involve a series of steps (A to B, B to C, C to D, etc). Drugs can theoretically affect any of these steps. For example, antidepressants can stop the metabolism of a neurotransmitter or block its reuptake into a neuron where it does not help a patient. Anti-arthritis medications can stop the production of prostaglandins (which cause inflammation), block signaling proteins that encourage inflammation, or directly block immune cells that cause inflammation.

Naturally the question arises "why does a particular drug cause X? Receptors control specific biological functions. The combination of a drug's shape and the particular atoms it has determines its characteristics. In short, a drug's overall structure determines which receptor(s) it binds with; which receptors it binds with determines its effects - both its intended effect and side-effects. Many different receptors have similar shapes and sizes, this allows a single drug to bind with different receptors causing a variety of effects.

Just as a particular key causes a conformational change inside a particular lock, allowing a doorknob to turn, agonist-drugs cause conformational changes in transmembrane cellular receptors; these conformational changes initiate a signaling cascade or open an ion-channel. Antagonist-drugs bind with the same receptor, but do not initiate a signaling cascade. Why the difference? Receptors have binding sites. These binding sites have various atoms arranged in a specific way. Agonist-drugs are physically shaped so their atoms physically align, either perfectly or nearly perfectly, with most or all of the atoms in the binding site, thus changing the shape of the receptor, thus initiating a signaling cascade or opening an ion-channel. Antagonist drugs are shaped in such a way that some of their atoms align with the atoms of the binding site, enough for the antagonist to bind with the binding site, but not enough to cause the conformational change needed to initiate a signaling cascade or open an ion-channel.

Drug receptors exist in many different forms. Drug receptors could be transmembrane cellular receptors, active sites of enzymes, extracellular proteins, intracellular proteins, DNA, neurotransmitter transporters, or other molecules. Receptors help control specific functions, such as regulating blood sugar and blood pressure.

A drug's ability to cause a biological result depends not just on its shape, but also the dose. For example nicotine, at low doses, stimulates breathing by stimulating the receptors of the aortic and carotid bodies. However, at higher doses, nicotine blocks receptors controlling nerve conduction to the muscles controlling breathing, potentially causing paralysis of these muscles and death.

PHARMACODYNAMICS AND PHARMACOKINETICS

Pharmacodynamics refers to what the drug does to the body; and how it does what it does; what changes in physiology or biochemistry occur as a result of the drug; and how did the drug cause these changes. The interaction between drugs and the human body is a two-way relationship. Just as drugs affect the body, the body affects drugs. What the body does to a drug is termed pharmacokinetics. Pharmacokinetics includes the absorption, distribution, metabolism, and excretion

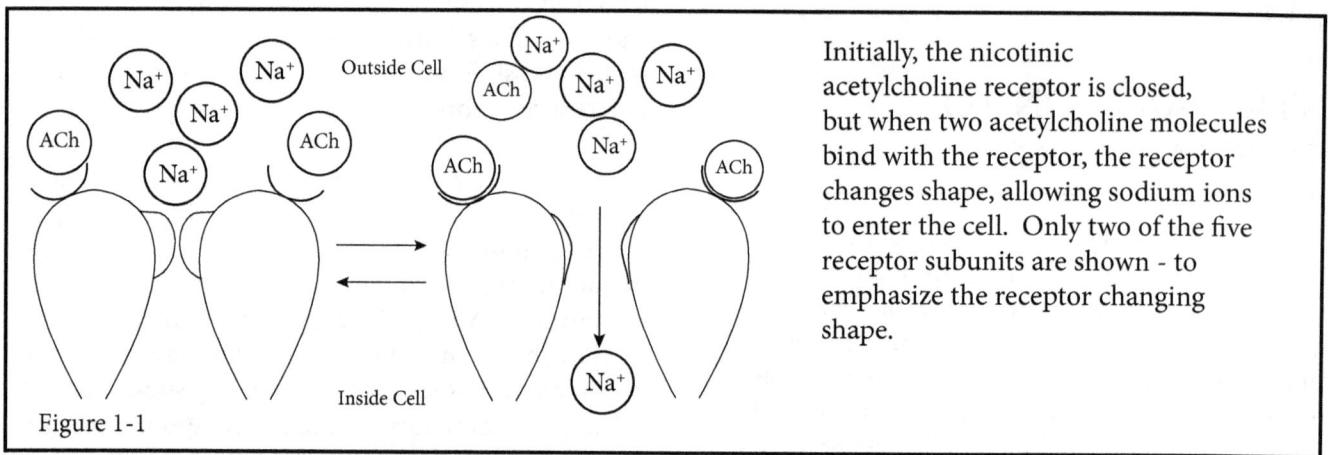

Initially, the nicotinic acetylcholine receptor is closed, but when two acetylcholine molecules bind with the receptor, the receptor changes shape, allowing sodium ions to enter the cell. Only two of the five receptor subunits are shown - to emphasize the receptor changing shape.

Figure 1-1

of drugs. Pharmacodynamics encompasses the therapeutic benefits of drugs and the adverse effects of drugs.

AGONISTS, ANTAGONISTS, AND RECEPTORS

Receptors, in general, have several important characteristics. Cellular receptors are proteins or glycoproteins (protein(s) combined with a sugar(s)). All receptors have a "primary binding site" where an endogenous substance binds; some also have an allosteric bind site, which is a distinct location from the primary binding site. An endogenous substance is something made by the body. Adrenalin and insulin are examples of endogenous substances. Most drugs bind at the primary binding site.

Drugs binding with cellular receptors are either agonists or antagonists. Agonists and antagonists can each be divided into smaller sub-categories, each with different characteristics. Full agonists produce 100% of a possible maximal response. Partial agonists produce less than a maximal response; some opioids fall into this category.

There are several different types of antagonists. Competitive antagonists block endogenous substances or agonists from binding with a receptor. When administered with an agonist, a competitive antagonist increases the dose of agonist needed to achieve a maximal response. Agonists and competitive antagonists bind and then unbind (dissociate) from a receptor, and the process repeats itself over and over. By giving enough agonist, when a competitive antagonist is present, the agonist can bind with enough receptors to achieve a maximal effect.

Non-competitive antagonists, at a certain dose, reduce the overall maximal effect of an agonist. Non-competitive antagonists stay bound long enough that they effectively preclude agonists from binding with the receptor.

Irreversible antagonists form covalent bonds with receptors that cannot be broken. Similar to a non-competitive antagonist, an irreversible antagonist reduces the overall maximal effect an agonist can achieve. At low doses, agonists can still achieve 100% maximal efficacy, however, as the amount of irreversible antagonist increases, agonists lose their ability to achieve a 100% maximal effect.

DRUG MECHANISMS OF ACTION

The vast majority of drugs work by binding with receptors or enzymes (the active site of an enzyme is sometimes called a receptor). Cellular receptors can be either on the surface of a cell, in the cytoplasm of a cell, or in the nucleus of a cell. Drugs also bind with extracellular enzymes (acetylcholine esterase), or with intercellular signaling molecules (TNF-alpha). The phrase "drug targets" was coined to encompass these additional sites of action because they are not "receptors" in the historical sense of the word. Not all drugs work by binding with cellular receptors. Some drugs neutralize stomach acid. Others alter the osmotic pressure within the colon to allow for a bowel movement.

Types of Receptors and Drug Targets:

- Ion channels - sodium ion channels, calcium ion channels, and potassium ion channels
- Nuclear receptors - glucocorticoids
- G-protein linked receptors - beta blockers

- Transmembrane receptors associated with intracellular enzymes - tyrosine kinases
- Intracellular enzymes - warfarin
- Extracellular enzymes - acetylcholine esterase inhibitors, angiotensin-converting-enzyme inhibitors. (Drug targets).

Ultimately, agonist drugs that bind with cellular receptors work by causing receptors to change shape (or stay in their already activated shape) (antagonists do not necessarily need to alter a receptors shape to work).

The shape change can cause several different events. For example, changing the shape of a receptor may open or close an ion channel, or initiate one of several different "signal transduction pathways." These pathways involve various enzymes, proteins, cyclic nucleotides, ions, and other secondary messengers. Some secondary messengers are cyclic adenosine mono-phosphate (cAMP), cyclic guanosine mono-phosphate (cGMP), and inositol triphosphate.

ION CHANNELS

In some cells, the exchange of ions from outside to inside, and conversely, from inside to outside propagates nerve signals ("voltage-gated" sodium channels). In other cells, this exchange of ions from outside to inside, and, conversely, from inside to outside allows the cell and tissue to contract. For example, vascular tissue surrounding arteries requires the influx of Ca^{2+} ions to ultimately contract the artery and increase blood pressure. By blocking Ca^{2+} channels, amlodipine prevents Ca^{2+} ions from entering arteries, thus dilating the vessel.

NUCLEAR RECEPTORS

Glucocorticoids work by binding with nuclear receptors. Glucocorticoids enter cells and travel to the nucleus (with the aid of other molecules) where they alter gene expression, including increasing the production of lipocortins (proteins). Lipocortins decrease the production of eicosanoids by preventing phospholipase A_2 from converting phospholipids to arachidonic acid, a necessary precursor to inflammatory eicosanoids. Glucocorticoids have other effects as well.

G PROTEIN LINKED RECEPTORS

Cellular receptors associated with G proteins are the largest class of cellular receptors. "G protein" is short for "heterotrimeric GTP-binding proteins." G proteins have three pieces (hence "trimeric"), which are an alpha unit, beta unit, and gamma unit. Their name derives from its function of binding with guanosine diphosphate (GDP) or guanosine triphosphate (GTP).

G proteins are divided into five main classes: G-stimulatory (G_s), G-inhibitory (G_i), G_o (inhibits Ca^{2+} channels), $G_{12/13}$ (influence ion transporters), and G_q (phospholipase C activation).

When a G protein associated receptor binds with a drug, the receptor undergoes a change in shape allowing part of the receptor that is inside the cell to bind with a G protein; initially the G protein is bound with GDP; however, upon binding with the receptor, GTP displaces the GDP from the alpha subunit. Then the combined alpha subunit and GTP break apart from the combined beta and gamma subunit. The alpha subunit and GTP are now free to stimulate secondary messengers, the exact messenger depends on the exact subtype of G protein involved (sometimes they open ion channels). The combined beta and gamma subunit complex can also initiate biochemical cascades.

Beta agonists, used to treat asthma, bind with beta receptors (G-protein coupled) in the lungs and cause the enzyme adenyl cyclase to increase the production of cAMP. cAMP stimulates several other biological cascades, ultimately causing bronchodilation.

TRANSMEMBRANE RECEPTORS WORKING WITH INTRACELLULAR ENZYMES

These receptors can have an enzyme as part of their overall physical structure or work closely with an intracellular enzyme. This class of receptors includes receptor tyrosine kinases and tumor-necrosis-factor-alpha (TNF-alpha) receptors, among others. Growth factors or other signaling proteins bind to these receptors, usually causing cell growth or inflammation. Overall, these receptors regulate the phosphorylation and dephosphorylation of intracellular proteins. The phosphorylation of a protein changes the proteins shape, which then allows the protein to act as a messenger, usually transmitting signals to the cell's nucleus, controlling cell growth, cell differentiation, or inflammation.

Some mutations in receptor-kinase systems can cause extra phosphorylation, possibly leading to cancer or inflammatory diseases, such as rheumatoid arthritis. Recently drugs have been developed inhibiting this extra phosphorylation. For example, imatinib and dasatinib inhibit the mutant receptor tyrosine kinase

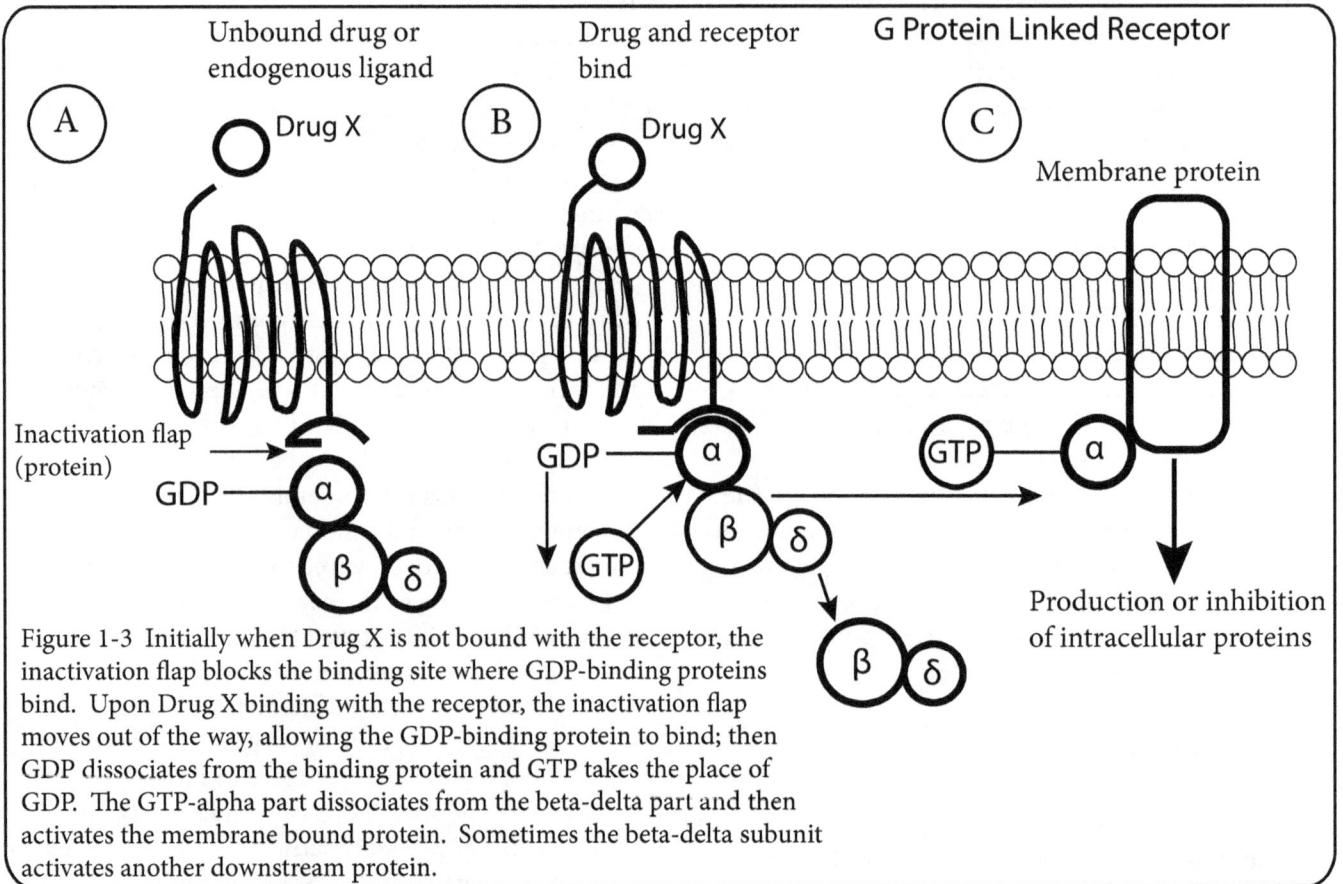

Figure 1-3 Initially when Drug X is not bound with the receptor, the inactivation flap blocks the binding site where GDP-binding proteins bind. Upon Drug X binding with the receptor, the inactivation flap moves out of the way, allowing the GDP-binding protein to bind; then GDP dissociates from the binding protein and GTP takes the place of GDP. The GTP-alpha part dissociates from the beta-delta part and then activates the membrane bound protein. Sometimes the beta-delta subunit activates another downstream protein.

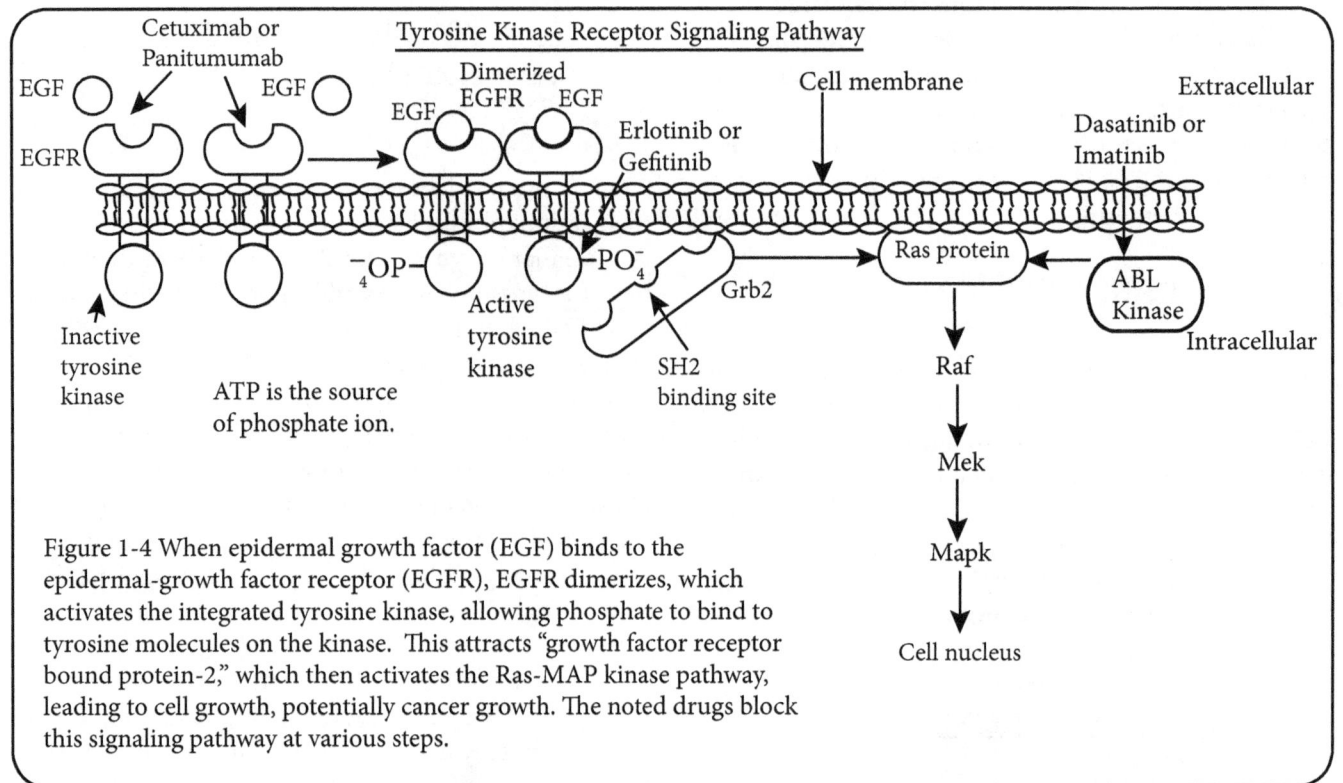

Figure 1-4 When epidermal growth factor (EGF) binds to the epidermal-growth factor receptor (EGFR), EGFR dimerizes, which activates the integrated tyrosine kinase, allowing phosphate to bind to tyrosine molecules on the kinase. This attracts "growth factor receptor bound protein-2," which then activates the Ras-MAP kinase pathway, leading to cell growth, potentially cancer growth. The noted drugs block this signaling pathway at various steps.

from spontaneously phosphorylating signaling proteins, thus reducing cell growth.

Additionally, several drugs inhibit TNF-alpha from binding with the TNF-alpha receptor, which would normally lead to the production of inflammatory mediators. Etanercept and adalimumab are examples of two TNF-alpha inhibitors.

INTRACELLULAR ENZYMES

Warfarin blocks the intracellular enzyme vitamin K reductase from producing the "reduced" form of vitamin K. The reduced form of vitamin K is necessary to produce circulating forms of coagulation factors II,VI, IX, and X, which are needed so blood clots can form when needed.

Blood clotting, in part, depends on coagulation factors II, VII, IX, and X. As proteins, they are synthesized on ribosomes. After leaving the ribosome, they still need to be transformed (carboxylated) before they can be released into the blood, waiting to form blood clots. The enzyme gamma-glutamyl carboxylase adds carboxyl groups to factors II, VII, IX, and X, transforming them into their final circulating forms in the blood, waiting for when they are needed to form a clot (which requires binding with Ca^{2+} ions). Gamma-glutamyl carboxylase needs (depends on) the reduced form of vitamin K so it can transform (carboxylate) factors II,VII, IX, and X to their circulating forms in the blood. Warfarin blocks the enzyme vitamin K reductase from producing the reduced form of vitamin K. The "oxidized" form of vitamin K is produced when gamma-glutamyl carboxylase adds carboxyl groups to coagulation factors II, VII, IX, and X. Then vitamin K reductase reforms the reduced form of vitamin K from the oxidized form of vitamin K; in other words, vitamin K is constantly circling between a reduced form and oxidized form, and wafarin blocks the regeneration of the reduced form of vitamin K.

EXTRACELLULAR ENZYMES

Extracellular enzymes function as drug-receptors for several drug classes. The extracellular enzyme acetylcholinesterase metabolizes acetylcholine, after acetylcholine has been released from a nerve ending; some drugs block acetylcholinesterase. Additionally, the extracellular enzyme angiotensin converting enzyme (ACE) converts angiotensin I to angiotensin II, a peptide the body uses to increase blood pressure. ACE-inhibitors prevent ACE from converting angioten-

sin I to angiotensin II.

GRADED DOSE-RESPONSE CURVES

Graded dose-response graphs tell you what happens in one particular person. Graded dose-response relationships tell you that as you increase the dose in a particular individual you increase the effect, up to a certain point, where the effect does not increase anymore because there can only be so many receptors or enzymes to bind with. As a practical significance, after a certain point, there is no benefit to further increasing the dose. Graded dose response curves are important to determine a general idea of an appropriate dose. However, quantal dose response curves generate much more clinically useful data. As a practical matter, you only see the end result of the quantal dose response curve in package inserts under the dosing section. See Figure 1-5 below.

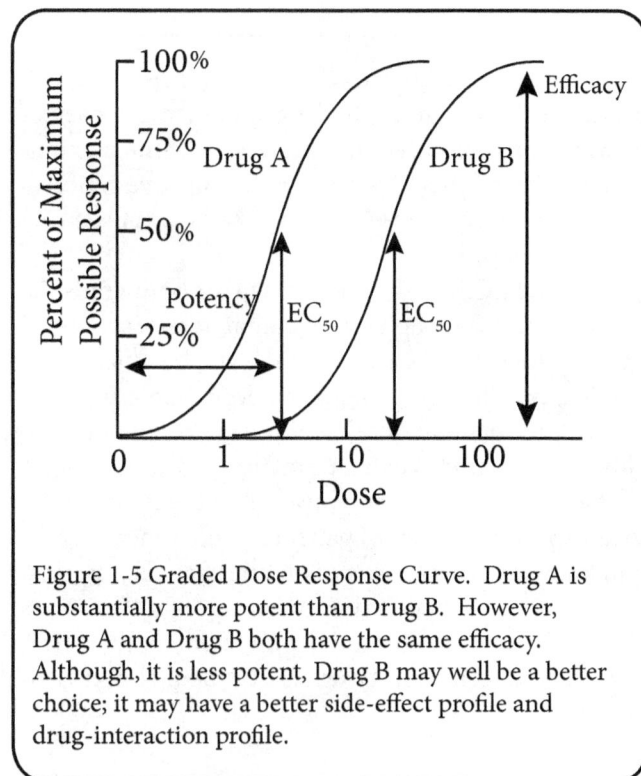

Figure 1-5 Graded Dose Response Curve. Drug A is substantially more potent than Drug B. However, Drug A and Drug B both have the same efficacy. Although, it is less potent, Drug B may well be a better choice; it may have a better side-effect profile and drug-interaction profile.

QUANTAL DOSE RESPONSE CURVES

Quantal dose-response relationships tell you that different people require different amounts of a drug to achieve the same effect. For example, out of 100 people, 10 people may need 1 mg of a sleeping drug to fall asleep; 30 people may need 3 mg to fall asleep and so on. Quantal dose-response curves tell us the dose at which 50% of patients have a therapeutic response (ED_{50}). The ED_{50} is used to help determine appropriate doses. See Figure 1-6.

EFFICACY

How well an agonist activates a receptor is called **efficacy**. Efficacy is the magnitude of a drug's affect on the body. How well a drug binds to a receptor and stays bound to the receptor is called **affinity**. Agonists and antagonists both have affinity for the receptors they bind with. However, only agonists activate receptors, and, therefore, only agonists have efficacy.

Antagonists do not have efficacy, meaning they do not activate the receptor, but this does not mean that antagonists do not have therapeutic value. Beta blockers are antagonists that provide therapeutic value by reducing blood pressure and heart rate.

POTENCY

Potency is how much of a drug is needed to produce a chosen effect. In drug studies, the chosen effect is the dose required to achieve 50% of the maximal possible effect. This is referred to as "effective concentration for 50% response" (EC_{50}). The EC_{50} is used to compare drugs.

The EC_{50} can be determined for both graded dose-response graphs and quantal dose-response graphs. However, the EC_{50} for each will be different. The EC_{50} is called ED_{50} in quantal dose-response graphs. The ED_{50} for quantal dose-response curves provides you with clinically useful data. Knowing the dose needed of a blood pressure drug to lower blood pressure by a certain amount in 50% of patients is more meaningful than knowing what happened in one particular person.

Figure 1-5 compares two drugs of differing potencies. Drug A is substantially more potent than Drug B - as can be seen from Drug A's EC_{50} being lower than Drug B's EC_{50}.

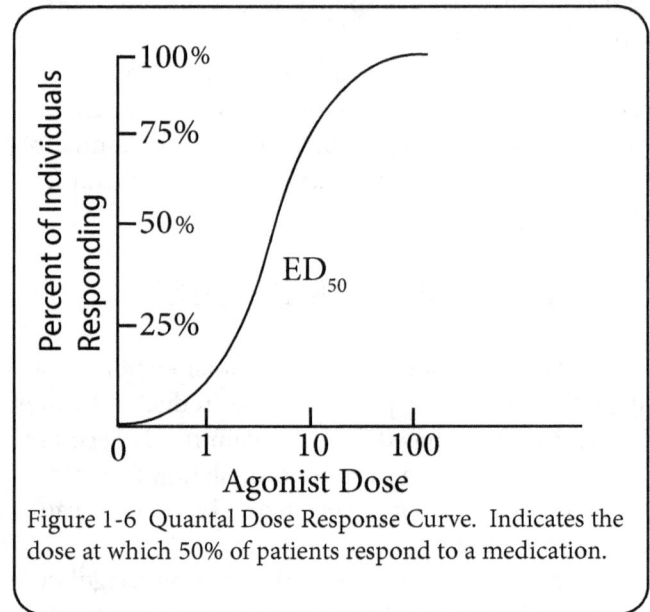

Figure 1-6 Quantal Dose Response Curve. Indicates the dose at which 50% of patients respond to a medication.

THERAPEUTIC WINDOW

Drugs at too low of a plasma concentration produce no effect. Drugs at too high of a plasma concentration may produce adverse effects. The range between too low a concentration and too high a concentration is known as the "therapeutic window". Clinicians need to know what these ranges are to safely and effectively prescribe medications. Researchers determine these ranges during clinical drug development trials; clinicians refine these ranges as clinical experience accumulates; some patients experience a clinical response at a much lower dose than the window would suggest. Further, some patients can handle, without adverse effects, doses much higher than the window would suggest.

THERAPEUTIC INDEX

The "therapeutic index" assesses the relative safety of a drug. Researchers determine the median lethal dose in laboratory animals (LD50) and divide it by the ED_{50} in humans to obtain the therapeutic index. From a clinical perspective, the bigger the number the better. If you need a high dose to cause death and a small dose to produce beneficial effects, then you have a wide range of safe plasma concentrations. Using a lethal dose in animals does not always correlate well with what happens in humans.

Consequently, researchers developed a new ratio to assess the safety of drugs. Researchers determine the dose or plasma concentration causing toxic results in 50% of a population (TD50) and divide it by the ED_{50} - this quotient is also referred to as a therapeutic index (TI) (also called the "therapeutic ratio). Remember, these definitions are based on what happens in the population; some people experience adverse effects at lower plasma concentration than others.

AGONISTS AND ANTAGONISTS GIVEN TOGETHER

At times, agonists and antagonists are used together in a clinical setting. This commonly occurs when clinicians are trying to treat overdoses. They are also given together in research settings to help determine a drug's mechanism of action.

A competitive antagonist increases the dose of agonist needed to achieve the EC_{50}. This is because an agonist normally has unopposed access to all of its receptors, but a competitive antagonist, intermittently blocks some of the receptors; because there a less receptors available to the agonist, its takes more agonist to bind the same number of receptors needed to achieve the EC_{50}. A competitive antagonist does not reduce an agonist's overall efficacy. In contrast, a non-competitive (irreversible) antagonist reduces the overall efficacy of an agonist.

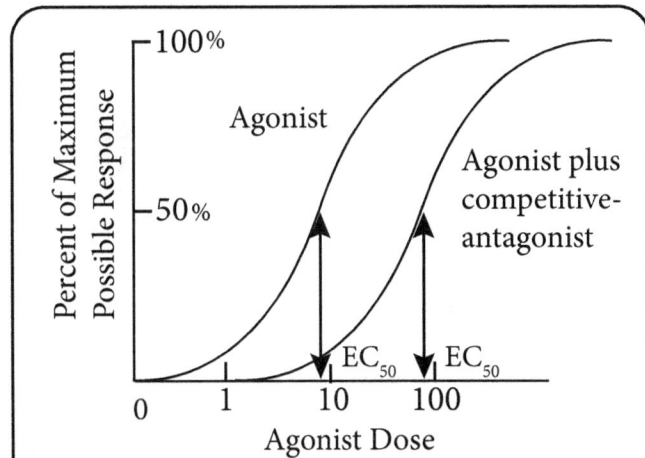

Figure 1-7 When a competitive antagonist is administered with an agonist, a higher dose of agonist is required to achieve 50% of the maximum possible response. The antagonist competes with the agonist for receptor binding sites, thus increasing the dose of agonist needed to achieve 50% of the maximum possible response.

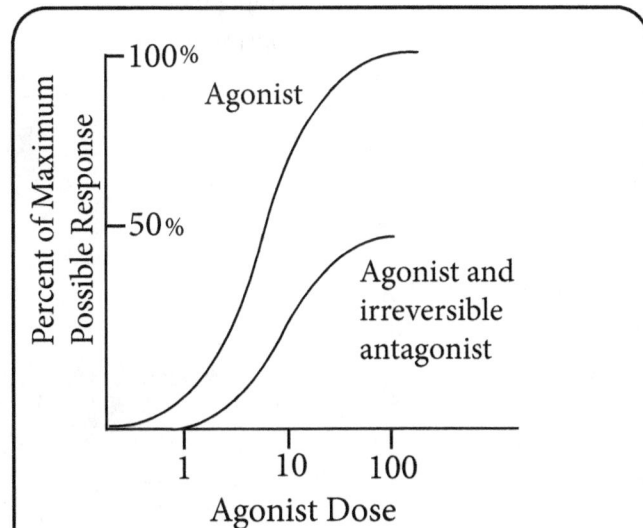

Figure 1-8 An irreversible antagonist covalently binds with receptors, thus reducing the number of available receptors the agonist can bind with, thus reducing the overall maximal effect of the agonist.

CHAPTER 2

INTRODUCTION TO PHARMACOKINETICS

Pharmacokinetics addresses the absorption, distribution, metabolism, and excretion of drugs - i.e., what the body does to the drug. How drugs pass through cell membranes influences these processes.

DRUG PASSAGE THROUGH CELL MEMBRANES

Most drugs must pass through cell membranes to reach their sites of action. Cell membranes are phospholipid bilayers; the exterior and interior surfaces are hydrophilic (water loving) and the interior portion of the phospholipid bilayer is hydrophobic. Cell membranes have aqueous channels (made of proteins) and transmembrane carrier proteins (transporters), both allow drugs into cells. Drugs can cross the phospholipid bilayer in several different ways:

1. Passive diffusion
2. Aqueous diffusion
3. Facilitated diffusion
4. Active transport - organic anion transporters (OAT); organic cation transporters (OCT); MDR1 (P-glycoprotein)
5. Endocytosis

Passive diffusion is when a drug simply diffuses through the lipid bilayer. Many drugs, such as steroids, passively diffuse through cell membranes. Passive diffusion occurs down a concentration gradient. The amount of passive diffusion depends on the difference in drug concentration between outside the cell and inside, the permeability coefficient of the membrane, the area of the cell membrane, and inversely related to the membrane's thickness.

Aqueous diffusion is the movement of a water soluble drug through transmembrane protein channels, which were designed for the diffusion of water into and out of cells. Small drugs are able to enter cells this way. Aqueous diffusion occurs down a concentration gradient.

Facilitated diffusion describes the process of a transmembrane carrier protein (transporter) moving a drug from outside to inside or inside to outside without the use of energy. Facilitated diffusion involves drug movement with their concentration gradient, and hence does not require energy.

Active transport describes the process of transmembrane carrier proteins using energy to move drugs from outside the cell to inside the cell, or vice-versa. Active transport is divided into two categories, *primary active transport* and *secondary active transport*. Primary active transport uses adenosine triphosphate (ATP) as its energy source, and secondary active transport uses the energy inherently stored in concentration gradients (more ionic solute on one side of a membrane than the other side). Active transport can move a drug against a concentration gradient. For example, P-glycoprotein, an efflux transporter, pumps digoxin, amongst

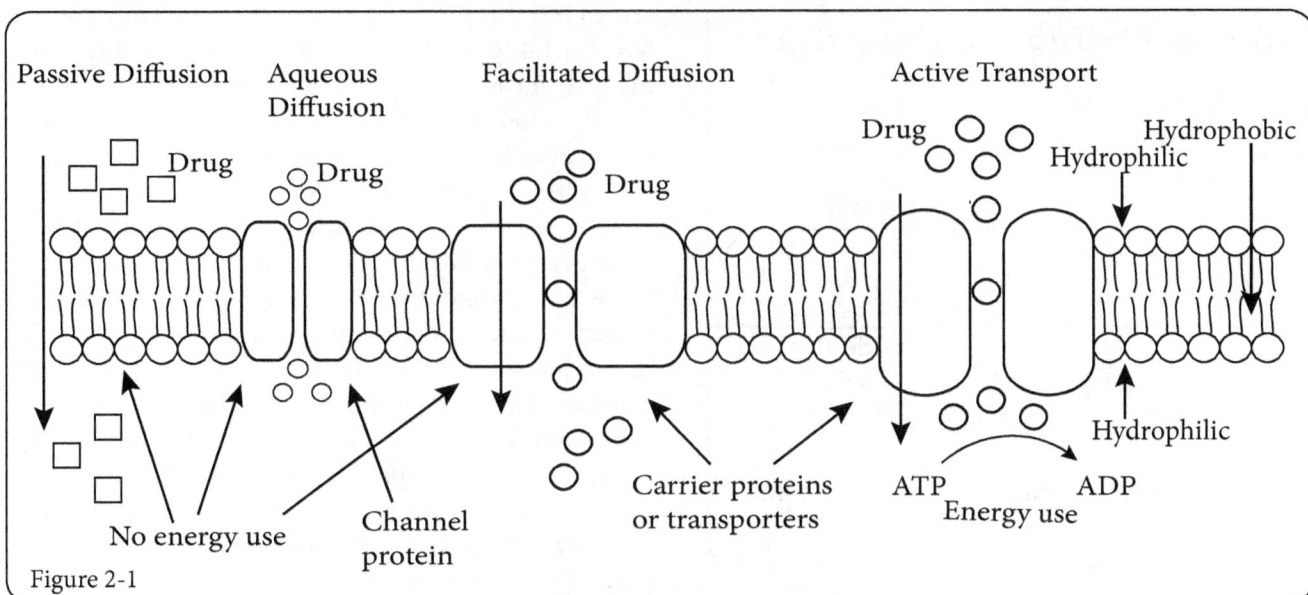

Figure 2-1

other drugs, out of intestinal cells back into the intestinal tract (lumen). P-glycoprotein also pumps some anticancer drugs out of cancer cells, thus conferring some cancer cells with resistance to some anticancer drugs.

Pinocytosis, a type of endocytosis, is how cells move large molecules into cells. Vitamin B12 enters cells through pinocytosis. In general, after a large molecule binds with receptors that regulate pinocytosis, (the necessity of binding with receptors indicates that only certain substances are allowed to enter a cell this way) the cell involutes or caves in on itself, forming a bubble around the molecule. After completely engulfing the molecule, the bubble releases the molecule into the cell.

ION-TRAPPING

The combination of a phospholipid bilayer and a difference in pH on each side of the bilayer creates "ion trapping" of drugs that are capable of being charged. Ion-trapping results when the ionized form of drug becomes trapped on one side of a cell membrane because of a difference in pH on each side of the membrane. For example, a weakly acidic drug will be protonated or un-ionized in the stomach because of the stomach's pH, but deprotonated or ionized in the plasma because of the plasma's pH. The un-ionized drug in the stomach may diffuse through the stomach into the plasma, however, the converse cannot happen. The weakly acidic drug will be ionized in the plasma

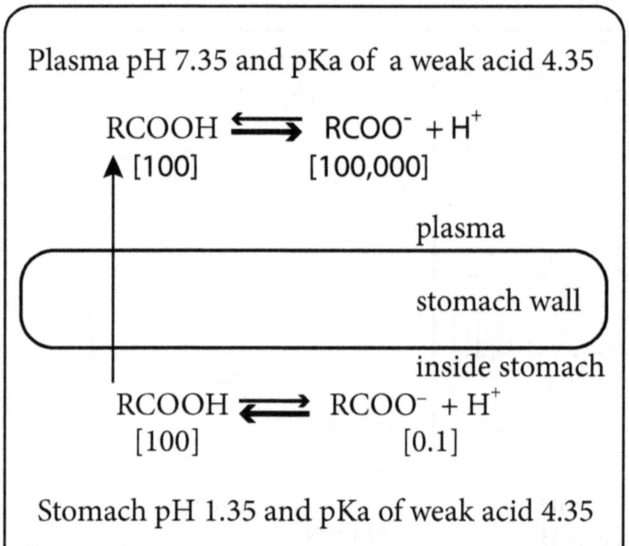

Plasma pH 7.35 and pKa of a weak acid 4.35

$$RCOOH \rightleftharpoons RCOO^- + H^+$$
$$[100] \qquad [100,000]$$

plasma

stomach wall

inside stomach

$$RCOOH \rightleftharpoons RCOO^- + H^+$$
$$[100] \qquad [0.1]$$

Stomach pH 1.35 and pKa of weak acid 4.35

Figure 2-2

and hence unable to diffuse through the stomach lining back into the stomach.

ABSORPTION AND BIOAVAILABILITY

Factors affecting absorption and bioavailability:

1) Route of administration
2) Dosage Form
3) Ionization of drug at physiological pH
4) Lipophilicity of drug
5) Rate of blood flow to intestinal tract
6) Overall health of intestinal tract
7) Food
8) Other drugs

For orally administered drugs (swallowed, not sublingual), **absorption** is how much drug passes through intestinal cells and enters the blood stream for delivery to the liver. **Bioavailability** is how much drug reaches the general circulation after passing through the liver. Because the liver metabolizes drugs, not all of an absorbed drug actually reaches the general circulation; this means that absorption and bioavailability are generally not equal. Bioavailability depends on the extent of absorption, route of administration and a patient's ability to metabolize a drug. Intravenously administered drugs have 100% bioavailability because they do not initially pass through the liver.

Liquid dosage forms may absorb better than tablets or capsules. "Binders," which are similar to glues, hold tablets together. Sometimes these binders prevent tablets from completely dissolving in the stomach and/or intestinal tract, thus limiting absorption and bioavailability. Ordinary gelatin capsules readily and easily dissolve in stomach acid.

Weak-acid drugs may be absorbed by a combination of diffusion and/or transport by organic anion transporters. Weak-acids are partially ionized in the upper intestinal tract. Non-ionized drug molecules diffuse through the large intestinal surface area. As those non-ionized drug molecules pass into the bloodstream, a certain amount of the ionized drug molecules (in the intestinal tract) have to become non-ionized as a matter of the laws of chemical equilibrium. Those newly non-ionized drug molecules then diffuse into the bloodstream and the process repeats itself.

Lipophilic (means a drug easily dissolves into fat) drugs absorb by passive diffusion. These drugs generally absorb well.

Patient specific factors affecting absorption

include: the rate of blood flow to the intestinal tract; overall health of intestinal tract; presence or lack of food in the intestinal tract; and disease states affecting intestinal cells. Diarrhea, regardless of the cause, limits absorption of not only nutrients but also drugs. Other patient factors include whether the patient is taking additional medications.

Some drugs prevent the absorption of other drugs. For example, antacids may bind with some antibiotics (fluoroquinolones) or thyroid medications, preventing their absorption. Some drugs inhibit drug transporters thus preventing the absorption of other drugs.

SUBLINGUAL ABSORPTION

Some drugs absorb sublingually (under the tongue). Nitroglycerin is commonly administered sublingually to treat angina. Drugs absorbed sublingually go directly into the blood stream via the superior vena cava and into the heart, bypassing the liver, initially. This is the rational for administering nitroglycerin sublingually during and emergency.

Suboxone, mirtazapine, ondansetron, and clonazepam, among others, can all be administered sublingually. Sublingual administration is useful for patients who have lost the ability to swallow, such as MS patients and elderly patients with Parkinson's disease or Alzheimer's disease.

INTRAVENOUS ADMINISTRATION

Absorption is not measured for intravenously administered drugs because they are injected directly into a vein or artery. Because the drug avoids first pass hepatic metabolism, bioavailability is considered to be 100%.

Sometimes the physical characteristics of a drug require IV administration. For example, the physical characteristics of proteins demand IV administration, if administered orally, the stomach digests them. Sometimes the situation requires IV administration; for example unconscious patients require IV administration.

The benefits of IV administration include complete bioavailability because the drug is injected into the blood. Onset of action is also within seconds to mere minutes. Intravenously administered drugs generally achieve a higher blood concentration than orally administered drugs; this is the reason why adverse reactions can be more intense or severe. If necessary, some intravenously administered drugs can be removed by dialysis.

SUBCUTANEOUS ABSORPTION

Subcutaneous administration may be used for drugs that cannot be taken orally because the stomach digests them, such as insulin and monoclonal antibodies. Insulin is usually administered subcutaneously, but may also be given intravenously in emergencies. IV administration of insulin does not last that long. Subcutaneous administration of insulin can last for as little as an hour to 24 hours depending on the formulation used. Subcutaneous administration is often used for other drugs and some vaccines.

INTRAMUSCULAR ABSORPTION

Intramuscularly administered drugs can rapidly absorb or slowly absorb depending on their formulation. Drugs in a water solution absorb into the blood stream fairly quickly; whereas, drugs in an oil base may persist for months. Antibiotics may absorb fairly quickly. In contrast, testosterone may stay in the muscle for two to four weeks. Further, medroxyprogesterone, a contraceptive, stays in muscle for three months. IM injections are also used for anti-psychotic drugs; compliance is often a problem in these patients.

PULMONARY ABSORPTION

Inhaled asthma and COPD drugs do not significantly enter the systemic circulation. However, drugs that are gases, anesthetics, or otherwise volatile may readily absorb through the lungs into the general circulation. Blood flows from the lungs directly to the heart, thus these drugs avoid hepatic first pass metabolism. Further, the large surface area of the lungs promotes rapid absorption.

TRANSDERMAL ABSORPTION

For the most part, transdermal absorption is used for a patient's convenience. In some cases, transdermal administration allows for better patient compliance because they do not have to remember to take a tablet several times a day. A transdermal patch may last for a full day (lidocaine) to a full week (some estrogen patches). Transdermal absorption is limited to lipophilic drugs. The amount of absorption depends on the surface area of the patch and the concentration of drug in the patch. Drugs administered transdermally avoid hepatic first pass metabolism.

TOPICAL ADMINISTRATION

Topically administered drugs, such as creams and ointments, readily absorb into the localized area needing treatment. Topically administered drugs are usually used for skin infections, eczema, and irritation from plants or animals (bee stings, animal bites). Triamcinolone and hydrocortisone are examples of topically administered drugs (hydrocortisone can also be administered orally).

TRANSPORTERS

Drug transporters and drug interactions influence absorption and bioavailability. Many drugs rely upon transporters to move them from the intestinal lumen to the blood stream, and from the blood stream into hepatocytes. (Hepatocytes are the functional cells of the liver that metabolize drugs.) In contrast, some transporters keep some drugs from being absorbed. For instance, the transporter P-glycoprotein (P-gp) pumps digoxin, a cardiac glycoside, out of intestinal cells and back into the intestinal lumen, preventing it from reaching the blood stream, thus reducing the amount of absorbed digoxin.

Some drugs can amplify the effect of P-gp by causing the body to produce more. For example, rifampin causes the body to produce additional P-gp; as a net result, the concurrent administration of rifampin, further decreases absorption of digoxin.

DISTRIBUTION

A drug's initial distribution depends on blood flow, and it's final distribution largely depends on its affinity for certain tissues (fat, muscle, etc) relative to its affinity for plasma proteins.

Initially, drugs distribute faster to organs with high blood flow relative to areas with low blood flow. Highly perfused areas include the liver, kidneys, and brain. Areas with relatively low blood flow include muscle, viscera, skin, and fat. Although distribution to fat cells may be slow, once there, lipophilic drugs may stay in fat cells for hours to days, or even weeks.

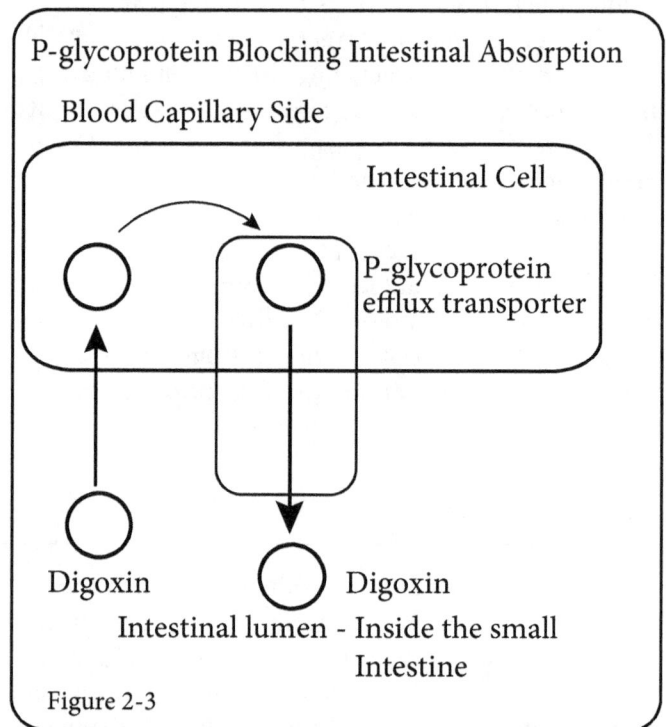

Figure 2-3

The **blood brain barrier** protects the human brain by limiting the distribution of drugs into it. Two independent tissues, capillaries and glial cells, form the blood brain barrier. Capillaries, normally have spaces between their endothelial cells, however, in the brain, these capillaries have "tight junctions," meaning there is not any space between the cells where a drug could pass through into the brain. Glial cells surround the capillaries, providing an extra layer of protection for the brain. As a consequence of the blood brain barrier, drugs must either be highly lipophilic, allowing them to diffuse through capillary and glial cells, or the drug must be a substrate for a transporter that can transport it into the brain. Benzodiazepines, highly lipophilic drugs, readily diffuse through the blood brain barrier. In contrast, many antibiotics and many anti-cancer drugs are neither lipophilic nor substrates for transporters, consequently, little, if any, of these drugs, enter the brain.

Some drugs distribute to bones and teeth; this is desirable in some circumstances and undesirable in other circumstances. For instance, the bisphosphonates, alendronate and sodium etidronate, preferentially distribute to bones, strengthening them by preventing the body from deconstructing bones through metabolism. In contrast, tetracycline undesirably distributes to teeth, discoloring them.

VOLUME OF DISTRIBUTION

The "volume of distribution" is to some extent an artificial concept. Its purpose is to tell you whether a drug prefers the blood or tissues; some drugs distribute evenly between the two. The volume of distribution indicates whether a drug stays in the plasma or distributes to the various tissues. The volume of distribution is based on the concentration of drug in the plasma. The volume of distribution represents the amount of fluid needed to dissolve the drug at the concentration in the plasma. This amount of fluid may equal the plasma volume or greatly exceed it. It may also exceed the total volume of water in the body. Volume of distribution is denoted by "V_d".

$$V_d = \text{Dose / Plasma Concentration}$$

The volume of distribution affects the half-life of a drug and the loading dose. As the volume of distribution increases, the half-life and loading dose proportionally increase.

Generally, the volume of distribution is low for drugs that are highly bound to plasma proteins and is high for drugs that readily dissolve in muscle or fat. Acidic and basic drugs tend to stay in the blood because acidic drugs bind to the plasma protein albumin, and basic drugs bind to alpha-1-acid glycoprotein.

Plasma protein levels influence drug distribution. Some diseases increase the amount of plasma proteins and some diseases decrease the amount of plasma proteins. Rheumatoid arthritis and burns may increase levels of alpha-1-acid glycoprotein, which would decrease free concentrations of basic drugs. Albumin levels usually decrease with chronic liver disease, resulting in higher levels of unbound drug.

A quick example. Suppose you inject 18 mg of drug into a 70 kg person; a 70 kg person has about 3 liters of plasma. Now take a blood sample and measure the concentration of drug in plasma. Suppose the drug has a concentration of 3 mg per liter. Based on that concentration, you would need 6 liters (18 mg/3 mg/L) of fluid to dissolve the drug. Well, the plasma has only 3 liters. Where is this other 3 liters of plasma? Well it does not exist. Rather, it means that 9 mg of drug (3 liters x 3 mg/L) is in the plasma and the other 9 mg has dissolved into various body tissues. In this example, one could conclude that the drug has equal affinity for plasma proteins as it does for tissue and fat cells.

METABOLISM

The body metabolizes most drugs to prevent them from harming the body and to reduce their presence in the body. Lipophilic drugs are especially metabolized. Renal tubules reabsorb lipophilic drugs from urine back into the general systemic circulation. Without metabolism, if a patient continued to take medication on a daily basis, the renal tubules would keep reabsorbing lipophilic drugs, then eventually dangerous concentrations of the drug would develop. Because of this, the body has developed the means to turn lipophilic drugs into hydrophilic drugs so the kidneys can effectively eliminate them in the urine. Metabolizing enzymes are mainly located in the intestinal tract and hepatocytes, but exist elsewhere, including the lungs and blood stream, among other locations.

Metabolism changes a drug's physical structure to accomplish either or both of the following goals: 1) inactivate the drug so it is no longer biologically active, and/or 2) make it more water soluble so the kidneys can more easily excrete the drug. Sometimes these goals are not accomplished. Sometimes metabolism creates an active metabolite out of an active drug (morphine).

The body has developed several different mechanisms for metabolizing drugs. Some of these include: phase I reactions, phase II reactions, enzymes metabolizing monoamines (sympathomimetic drugs), and enzymes metabolizing acetylcholine. The names "phase I" and "phase II" suggest that after a drug undergoes phase I metabolism, it then must undergo phase II metabolism; this is not true. A drug can undergo phase I metabolism without undergoing phase II metabolism; further, a drug can undergo phase II metabolism without undergoing phase I metabolism (acetaminophen). Finally, as expected, a drug can undergo phase I metabolism and then phase II metabolism.

PHASE I REACTIONS

Phase I reactions generally inactivate a drug. Phase I reactions generally occur through the cytochrome P 450 isoenzyme system; this is the primary means of metabolism. Phase I reactions may expose an existing functional group in the drug, or add a new functional group to the drug, usually making it more water soluble. Functional groups provide a place for Phase II reactions to attach other molecules. New functional groups are formed by oxidizing, reducing, or hydrolyzing the drug. There are several types of phase I reactions:

1. N-Dealkylation
2. O-Dealkylation
3. Aliphatic hydroxylation
4. Aromatic hydroxylation
5. N-Oxidation
6. S-Oxidation

PHASE II REACTIONS

Phase II reactions add a hydrophilic group to the drug or its metabolite from a phase I reaction. This polar group generally makes the drug or metabolite more water soluble and hence more easily excreted by the kidneys. Phase II reactions are handled by conjugating enzymes, including glutathione-S-transferases, UDP-glucuronosyltransferases, sulfotransferases, N-acetyltransferases, and methyltransferases. These enzymes usually transfer a hydrophilic group to the metabolite from the phase I reaction. These hydrophilic groups are sulfate groups, glucuronic acid groups, or glutathione. Phase II reactions may also add acetyl or methyl groups, which may make metabolites less water soluble. In general Phase II reactions inactivate drugs, however, important exceptions exist. For example, the liver metabolizes morphine into a glucuronide conjugate that is more biologically active than morphine.

PHARMACOKINETICS: DRUG INTERACTIONS

INDUCTION OF CYP450 ISOENZYMES

Some drugs induce the liver to produce more of certain CYP450 isoenzymes, resulting in faster metabolism of drugs subject to metabolism by that enzyme. For example, alcohol induces CYP450 isoenzymes. As a result, people who drink alcohol on a regular basis, produce more CYP450 isoenzymes than people who do not consume alcohol.

Phenytoin, a difficult drug to dose in many patients, is not only metabolized by CYP2C9, but also induces the production of CYP2C9. This increase in production of CYP2C9 depends on the dose of phenytoin, and the more phenytoin given means a bigger induction in its own metabolism. Many other drugs induce hepatic enzymes.

INHIBITION OF CYP450 ISOENZYMES

In contrast, some drugs inhibit CYP450 isoenzymes, resulting in slower metabolism of drugs that are metabolized by the inhibited enzyme. As an example, ketoconazole, a strong inhibitor of CYP 3A4, inhibits the metabolism of protease inhibitors, leading to increased plasma concentrations of protease inhibitors and side-effects; ketoconazole affects the metabolism of other drugs metabolized by CYP3A4 as well. Other drugs inhibiting CYP3A4 include erythromycin, cyclosporine A, nefazodone, and amiodarone. In particular, these drugs inhibit the metabolism of most anti-cholesterol drugs (simvastatin, atorvastatin, and lovastatin).

PLASMA PROTEIN BINDING INTERACTIONS

Drugs highly binding with plasma proteins (particularly albumin) can interact with other drugs that highly bind with plasma proteins. The practical consequence of this can be a severe or life-threatening drug interaction. Warfarin highly binds with albumin (about 99%); the slightest displacement from albumin by other drugs can dramatically increase the unbound ("free") concentration of drug in the plasma, which is the practical equivalent of an overdose. This makes it more difficult for the patient to stop bleeding once bleeding starts. See figure 2-4.

GASTROINTESTINAL INTERACTIONS

Additionally, some drugs interfere with the absorption of other drugs. For example, both sucralfate and cholestyramine limit the absorption of other drugs. Sucralfate should be administered two hours after other medications to eliminate the interaction. Prevent drug interactions by administering cholestyramine four hours after other medications.

EXCRETION

The kidneys excrete drugs to protect the body. The kidneys excrete drugs through glomerular filtration and tubular secretion. However, through a process called tubular reabsorption, the kidneys reabsorb drugs back into the blood from urine. Lipophilic drugs tend to be reabsorbed into the blood. Lipophilic drugs tend to be un-ionized. A drug's structure and the urine's pH determine whether it will be ionized or un-ionized in

Table 2-1 Summary of Major Drug-Drug Interactions			
CYP Subfamily	Inhibitors	Inducers	Substrates
1A2	Ciprofloxacin, fluvoxamine, oral contraceptives, cimetidine	Smoking relative to not smoking, montelukast, phenytoin	Theophylline, duloxe-tine, caffeine, tizanidine, warfarin
2C9	Amiodarone, fluconazole, metronidazole	Carbamazepine, rifampin	Warfarin, phenytoin
2D6	Bupropion, fluoxetine, paroxetine, quinidine	Unknown	Thioridazine, metopro-lol, venlafaxine, dextro-methorphan
3A4	Clarithromycin, amiodarone grapefruit juice, ketoconazole	Carbamazepine, phenyt-oin, rifampin, St. John's wort	Cyclosporine, tacrolim-us, simvastatin, fentanyl, alfentanil, quinidine, warfarin

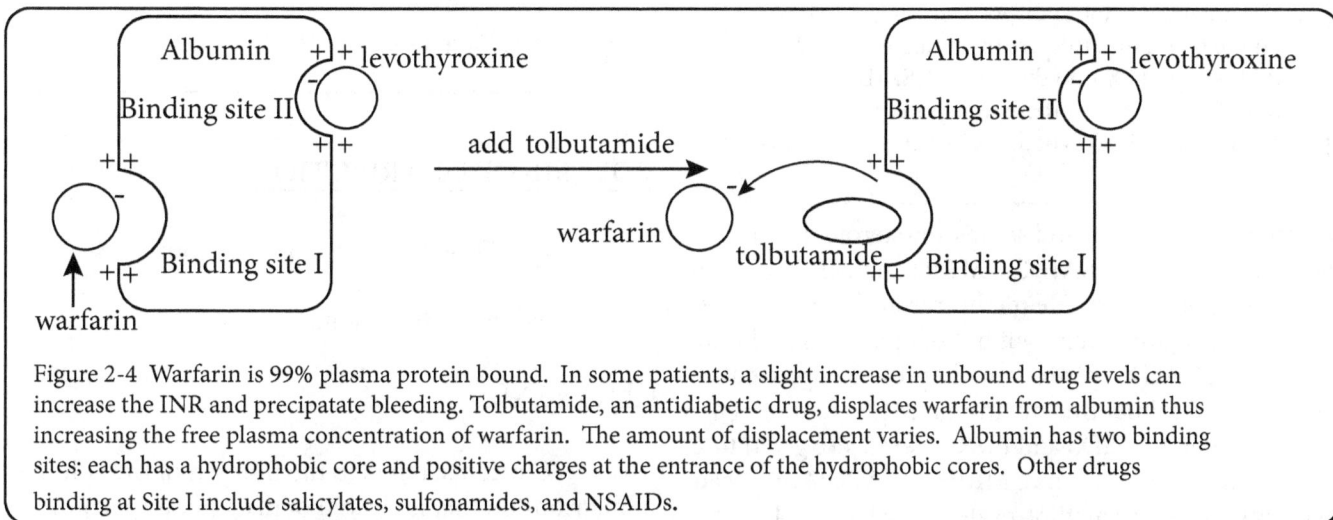

Figure 2-4 Warfarin is 99% plasma protein bound. In some patients, a slight increase in unbound drug levels can increase the INR and precipatate bleeding. Tolbutamide, an antidiabetic drug, displaces warfarin from albumin thus increasing the free plasma concentration of warfarin. The amount of displacement varies. Albumin has two binding sites; each has a hydrophobic core and positive charges at the entrance of the hydrophobic cores. Other drugs binding at Site I include salicylates, sulfonamides, and NSAIDs.

the urine.

Clinicians alkalinize or acidify the urine to cause the kidneys to more rapidly excrete ionized drugs during emergencies, usually overdoses, intentional or unintentional. Ionized drugs are easily excreted in the urine. Alkaline urine causes weak acid drugs to be ion-ized, and, therefore, excreted into the urine. Clinicians use sodium bicarbonate to alkalinize the urine. Con-versely, acidic urine causes weak bases to be ionized, and, therefore, excreted into the urine. Cranberry juice acidifies urine.

Just as other areas of the body have transporters moving drugs into and out of cells, so do the kidneys. Transporters help the kidneys excrete drugs and their metabolites. Organic anion-transporters (OATs) help the kidneys remove drugs with a negative charge (anions). Organic-cation transporters (OCTs) help the kidneys remove drugs with a positive charge (cations). Other transporters exist for uncharged drugs (MRPs).

Probenecid blocks OATs. OATs helps excrete penicillins. Thus, the concurrent administration of probenecid and penicillin increases penicillin plasma levels. Sometimes clinicians use this interaction to the patients advantage, allowing higher levels of penicillins to be achieved with lower doses.

P-gp pumps digoxin out of kidney cells and into the fluid becoming urine. However, inhibitors of P-gp prevent it from pumping digoxin out and into the urine. These inhibitors include: clarithromycin, ritona-vir, quinidine, spironolactone, vaspodar, and verapamil. When co-administered with digoxin, these inhibitors increase digoxin's blood concentration.

Inhibiting renal excretion of some drugs can cause death. Fatal drug interactions have occurred

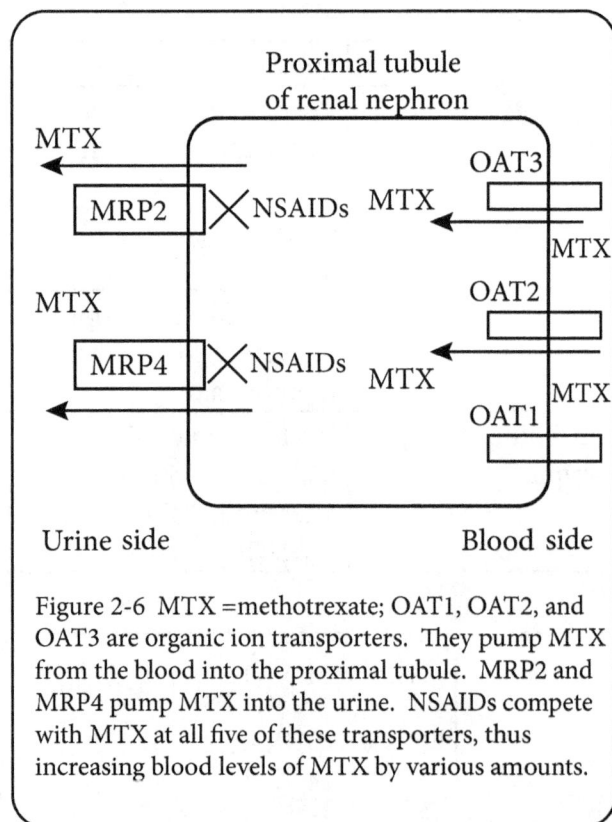

Figure 2-6 MTX =methotrexate; OAT1, OAT2, and OAT3 are organic ion transporters. They pump MTX from the blood into the proximal tubule. MRP2 and MRP4 pump MTX into the urine. NSAIDs compete with MTX at all five of these transporters, thus increasing blood levels of MTX by various amounts.

between methotrexate and some non-steroidal anti-inflammatory drugs (NSAIDS). MRP2 and MRP4 (two renal transporters) excrete methotrexate from the body by transporting or effluxing it out of renal cells and into the urine. NSAIDS (piroxicam, ibuprofen, naproxen, sulindac, and tolmentin, etc) inhibit MRP2 and MRP4.

When NSAIDS and methotrexate are given together, NSAID inhibition of MRP2 and MRP4 may lead to harmful levels of methotrexate in the blood. Use caution when using NSAIDS and methotrexate together, if at all.

ENTEROHEPATIC CYCLING

Hepatocytes use transporters to efflux (move a drug from inside a cell to outside the cell) drugs and drug metabolites into bile. While in bile, these drugs and metabolites pass through the intestinal tract to either leave the body as part of stool or to be reabsorbed from the GI tract, a second time, back into the hepatic circulation. These reabsorbed drugs have a second chance to enter the general circulation or be excreted back into bile and the intestinal tract a second time. This is enterohepatic recycling and is the reason why some drugs have long half-lives. Drugs that are not excreted in the bile, enter the general circulation.

ELIMINATION OF DRUGS

The body "eliminates" most drugs on a "first-order" basis. First-order elimination means the body eliminates a constant <u>percentage</u> of the amount of drug, in the body, per unit time. A constant percentage of a continuously decreasing amount of drug means that a <u>smaller amount</u> of drug is eliminated per each successive unit of time. In contrast, in limited situations, the body eliminates drugs on a "zero-order" basis. Zero-order means the body eliminates a <u>constant amount</u> of drug per unit time. The word "elimination" includes metabolism, urinary excretion, and biliary excretion. A drug could be "eliminated" by metabolism, but the metabolite may still physically be in the body. At high doses, aspirin and phenytoin are eliminated on a zero-order basis. Ethanol is eliminated on a zero-order basis.

CALCULATIONS

VOLUME OF DISTRIBUTION

V_d = Dose / Plasma Concentration

See above discussion.

CLEARANCE

Clearance refers to the fraction of the volume of distribution that is cleared of drug per a specified amount of time. Clearance includes hepatic clearance and renal clearance. Clearance has units of volume per time and is abbreviated as "Cl."

$Cl = k_{el} \times V_d$

The letter "k_{el}" represents the fraction of drug removed by the body per specified amount of time. K_{el} is the slope of the line formed when the log of the plasma concentration is graphed versus time. On semi-log graph paper, this produces a straight line, and K_{el} is the slope (see graph).

Through algebra, clearance can also be defined as:

Cl = rate of elimination / C_p

This second equation results from rearranging

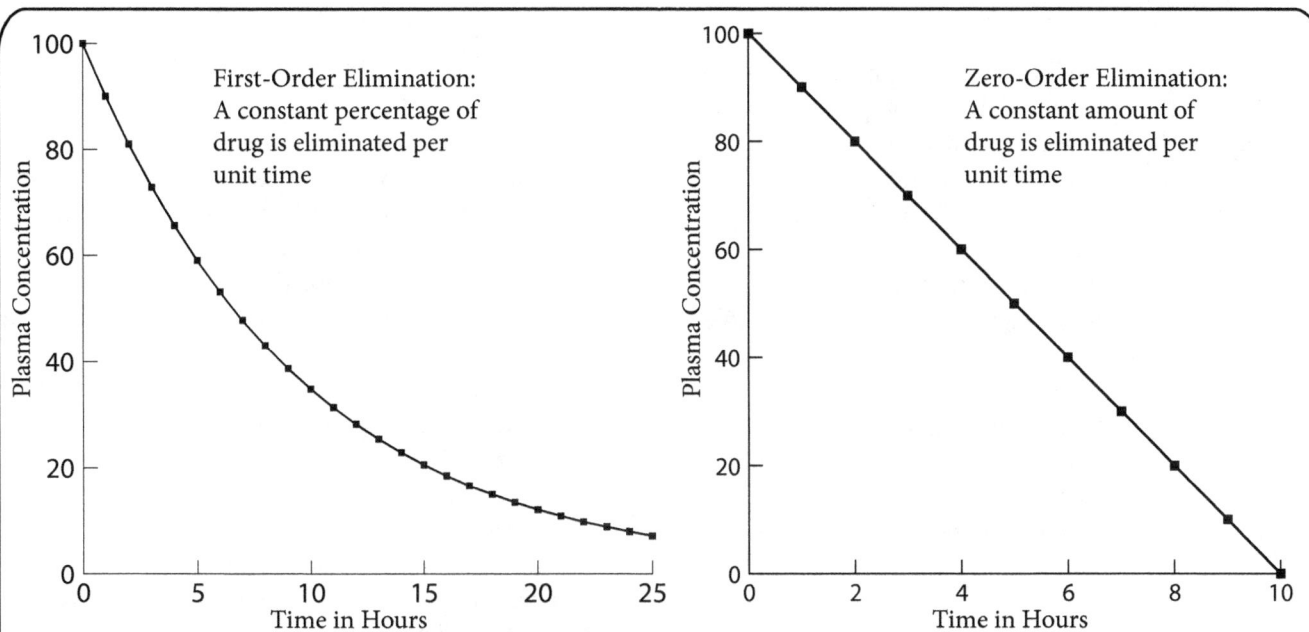

Figure 2-7 For most drugs, at normal doses, the body eliminates a certain percentage of drug per unit time (one hour, or so, it does not really matter what interval you pick). The percentage factor gives rise to the characteristic curve of these graphs. As the amount of drug in the body decreases, the amount eliminated also decreases, so although the data points move to the right a constant amount, they move downward by a decreasing amount - producing the curve. Consider the simplest scenario of a drug that is only renally eliminated. It's elimination depends on the probability of it contacting a renal transporter to remove it from the blood and deposit it in the urine. The probability of contacting a transporter directly depends on the amount of drug in the plasma passing through the kidneys.

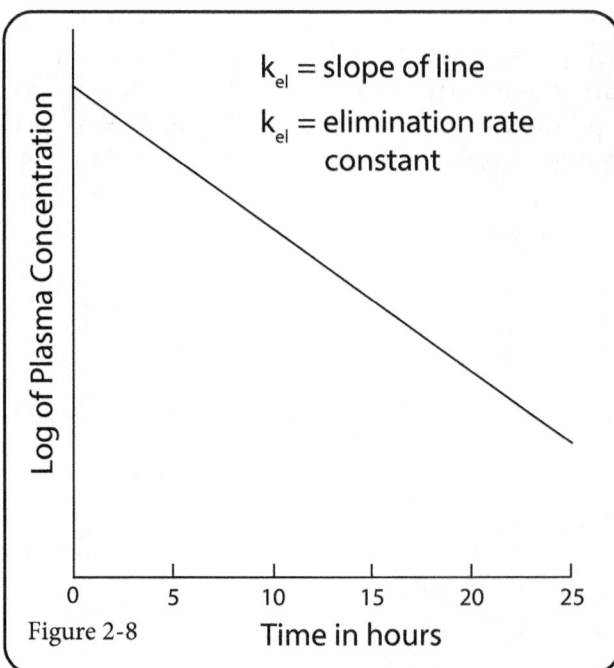

Figure 2-8

k_{el} = slope of line

k_{el} = elimination rate constant

and substituting factors into the first equation.

During drug development studies, clearance is measured in healthy subjects. Clearance is constant in patients with normal renal, hepatic, and cardiac function. However, clearance can change substantially in patients with decreased cardiac, renal, and/or liver function. Creatine clearance is used as a measure of renal function. Drugs relying on kidney function for clearance, should have their dosages decreased when creatine clearance is decreased. Patients with decreased hepatic function or cardiac function also require decreased doses.

HALF-LIFE

The elimination half-life of a drug is the amount of time needed for the plasma concentration to decrease by one-half or fifty percent. Half-life depends on the volume of distribution and clearance. For drugs following first order kinetics and considering the body as a single compartment, the $t_{1/2}$ is calculated as:

$$t_{1/2} = 0.693 \times V_d / Cl$$

The half-life tells us how long it will take for a drug to reach steady state and how long it will take for the body to eliminate a drug. Theoretically, it takes an infinite amount of time to reach steady state, however, as a practical matter, it is considered to be about 4 half-lives. At four half-lives, a drug will achieve 93.75% of its steady state plasma concentration. The 6.25% difference is not large enough to produce a noticeable therapeutic difference. Similarly, it takes forever to completely eliminate a drug, however, after about 4 half-lives, the little remaining drug is insignificant.

The half-life of a drug changes as a patient's kidney, hepatic, and/or cardiac function changes. A decrease in any of these can increase a drug's half-life.

STEADY STATE

As a general principle, while a patient is being treated, drug levels should remain as constant as possible. Steady-state is when the rate of drug dosing equals the rate of drug elimination. For a constant IV infusion, plasma concentration levels would be the same at all times. For oral dosing, the steady-state level is the average of the peak plasma concentration and the trough plasma concentration level; the amount of drug in the body stays the same between each dosing interval.

The time to reach steady-state cannot be reduced by increasing the infusion rate. Increasing the infusion rate simply increases the plasma concentration at steady-state. If a desired plasma concentration needs to be achieved quickly, consider using an IV bolus dose as opposed to increasing the rate of infusion.

MAINTENANCE DOSING

Maintenance dosing maintains a steady-state plasma drug concentration. Maintenance dosing is based on the principle that the rate of administration must equal the rate of elimination. Maintenance dosing depends on clearance (Cl) and the steady-state concentration (C_{SS}) as follows:

Maintenance dose = Cl x C_{SS}

or, stated in units:

$$\frac{mg}{hour} = \frac{volume}{hour} \times \frac{mg}{volume}$$

After calculating the dose per hour needed to maintain the steady-state plasma concentration, you should calculate the total daily dose by multiplying by 24 hours. Depending on the drug, you might administer the total daily dose in one dose, or divide it into two to four doses depending on the half-life of the drug and the width of the **therapeutic window**.

For orally administered drugs, the maintenance dose may need to be adjusted for bioavailability. Divide the calculated maintenance dose by the known bioavailability of the drug to adjust for bioavailability problems. As a practical matter, you will not be able to achieve an exact dose with tablets or capsules, however, since most drugs have a wide therapeutic window, it is okay to administer a slightly higher or lower dose for most patients with normal renal and kidney function.

LOADING DOSE

The loading dose is the dose needed to quickly achieve a chosen plasma concentration; it can be used for many drugs, including antibiotics. Without a loading dose, it would take four half-lives to reach a practical steady-state plasma concentration. For most out-patients, waiting four half-lives does not pose any problem to the patient. For hospitalized patients, quickly achieving a therapeutic steady-state plasma concentration may be a necessity. The loading dose is simply the volume of distribution (V_d) multiplied by the steady-state plasma concentration (C_{SS}).

Loading dose = V_d x C_{SS}

CHAPTER 3

CHOLINERGIC AND ANTICHOLINERGIC DRUGS

Cholinergic Drugs		Anticholinergic Drugs	
Direct acting drugs bind directly with acetylcholine receptors (called muscarinic or nicotinic receptors)	Indirect acting drugs inhibit acetylcholinesterase	Muscarinic Antagonists: block acetylcholine at muscarinic receptors	Nicotinic Antagonists: Block acetylcholine at nicotinic receptors in skeletal muscle

Acetylcholine
Bethanechol
Carbachol
Methacholine
Nicotine
Pilocarpine
Varenicline
	Echothiophate Iodide
	Edrophonium
	Malathion
	Neostigmine
	Physostigmine
	Pyridostigmine
	Malathion
		Atropine
		Benztropine
		Dicyclomine
		Flavoxate
		Glycopyrrolate
		Homatropine
		Oxybutynin
		Scopolamine
		Tolterodine
		Trihexyphenidyl
			1) Neuromuscular blockers:
			   1A) Depolarizing blockers: Succinylcholine
			
			   1B) Non-depolarizing blockers: Tubocurarine
			
			2) Ganglionic blockers: no longer clinically used

Cholinergic drugs have effects that are similar to acetylcholine. Anticholinergic drugs antagonize the effects of acetylcholine. Acetylcholine is a neurotransmitter that plays an important role in the peripheral nervous system. First, a brief review of the peripheral nervous system.

The peripheral nervous system consists of the autonomic nervous system and somatic nervous system. The somatic nervous system controls skeletal muscles. The autonomic nervous system divides into the sympathetic nervous system and parasympathetic nervous system. The ANS controls involuntary bodily functions such as digestion, pupil reflexes, breathing, heart rate, blood pressure, and many others. Most organs or non-skeletal muscle are innervated by both sympathetic and parasympathetic nerves. This means that organs and tissues have drug receptors for both systems. When receptors for one system are blocked, then the other system has more influence over that organ or tissue. For example, if you block beta receptors (sympathetic system) in the lungs, then the natural parasympathetic tone to the lungs causes bronchoconstriction.

The sympathetic system controls the 'flight or fight' response. The sympathetic system increases heart rate, dilates bronchi, and decreases gastrointestinal motility. The parasympathetic system decreases heart rate, decreases blood pressure, increases gastrointestinal secretions, increases gastrointestinal motility, constricts the pupils, empties the bladder, and empties the rectum.

The sympathetic and parasympathetic systems each use two separate neurons to send messages from the spinal cord to an organ or muscle. The space between the two neurons is called a synapse. The neuron before the synapse and closer to the spinal cord is called the "presynaptic neuron." The neuron after the synapse and closer to the end organ or muscle is called the "post-synaptic neuron." The locations where many presynaptic and post-synaptic neurons meet is called a ganglion. Sympathetic ganglia are located next to the spinal cord. Parasympathetic ganglia are spread throughout the body.

Control of tissues, muscles, and organs occurs in a step wise fashion for both the parasympathetic and sympathetic systems. In an overly generalized explanation, starting from the spinal cord, the presynaptic neuron releases a neurotransmitter across the synapse and binds with a receptor on the postsynaptic neuron. This causes biochemical changes to occur in the postsynaptic neuron. These changes propagate a nerve signal through the postsynaptic neuron towards the end

Tissue / Muscle / Organ	Parasympathetic System - Acetylcholine:	Sympathetic System - Norepinephrine:
Iris sphincter muscle	Contracts muscle causing miosis (pin point pupils); M_3 and M_2 receptor mediated	---
Iris radial muscle	---	Contracts muscle causing mydriasis (dilation); alpha$_1$ receptor mediated
Ciliary Muscle (eye muscle)	Contracts muscle for near vision; M_3 and M_2 receptor mediated	Relaxes muscle for far vision; beta$_2$ receptor mediated
Salivary Glands	Increases secretions; M_3 and M_2 mediated	Increases secretions but much less than parasympathetic system; alpha$_1$ mediated
Lungs Bronchial smooth muscle	Constricts airways; M_3 and M_2 mediated	Relaxes airways; beta$_2$ mediated
Bronchial glands	Increases secretions; M_3 and M_2 mediated	Decreases secretions alpha$_1$ mediated
Heart	Slows heart rate and decreases contractility; M_2 mediated	Increases heart rate and increases contractility; mostly beta$_1$ mediated but some beta$_2$
Intestinal Motility	Increases intestinal motility; M_3 and M_2 mediated	Decreases intestinal motility; alpha$_1$, alpha$_2$ beta$_1$, and beta$_2$ mediated
Intestinal Secretions	Increases secretions; M_3 and M_2 mediated	Decreases secretions; alpha$_2$ mediated
Sweat Glands	Parasympathetic system does not innervate sweat glands except palms of hands	Increases sweating (acetylcholine is the neurotransmitter)
Detrusor muscle of Bladder	Contracts detrusor muscle causing urination; M_3 receptor mediated	Relaxes detrusor muscle, allowing bladder to fill; beta$_2$ mediated
Urinary Sphincter	Relaxes sphincter muscle, allowing urine to pass; M_3 receptor mediated	Contracts sphincter muscle, preventing urination; alpha$_1$ mediated
Vascular Smooth Muscle	Not innervated by parasympathetic system	Increases blood pressure by constricting vascular smooth muscle; mostly alpha$_1$ mediated
Liver	--	Increases blood sugar by glycogenolysis and gluconeogenesis; alpha$_1$ and beta$_2$ mediated respectively

The parasympathetic nervous system uses acetylcholine as a neurotransmitter 1) at its ganglia, which is where its presynaptic and postsynaptic neurons meet, and 2) at the junction between the end of its postsynaptic neuron and effector cells (tissue, muscle, or organ). The sympathetic nervous system also uses acetylcholine at its ganglia, but uses norepinephrine at its effector cells, except sweat glands where its uses acetylcholine.

Preganglionic sympathetic neurons are short, and postganglionic sympathetic neurons are long. Preganglionic parasympathetic neurons are long, and postganglionic parasympathetic neurons are short, the exact opposite of the sympathetic system. This text uses "presynaptic" and "preganglionic" interchangeably.

organ, muscle, or tissue. When the signal reaches the end of the postsynaptic neuron, the signal causes the postsynaptic neuron to release its own neurotransmitter into the end organ, muscle, or tissue that it innervates. This could increase gastrointestinal tone, decrease heart rate, or dilate bronchioles, among other actions.

ACETYLCHOLINE

Acetylcholine affects many organs and muscles including the eyes, heart, lungs, smooth muscle of the genitourinary system, and skeletal muscle. Reveiw the corresponding table for a more detailed review of acetylcholine's actions. Acetylcholine is the principal neurotransmitter between presynaptic neurons and post-synaptic neurons of both the parasympathetic and sympathetic systems. Acetylcholine is also the principal neurotransmitter between parasympathetic post-ganglionic neurons and their effectors cells, such as the eye, lungs, heart, GI tract, bladder, and sweat glands. The sympathetic system uses acetylcholine at sweat glands. The somatic nervous system uses acetylcholine as a neurotransmitter at the neuromuscular junction.

Acetylcholinesterase is an enzyme that metabolizes acetylcholine in the synapse between two neurons or at the synapse between a postsynaptic neuron and the neuron's end-effector cells. Acetylcholinesterase inhibitors treat several different diseases, such as glaucoma, urinary retention, and paralytic ileus.

The names for acetylcholine receptors can be difficult to understand at first; this is because of how and when they were discovered. Acetylcholine binds with both muscarinic receptors and nicotinic receptors. The names "muscarinic" and "nicotinic" are used because researchers knew about muscarine (a chemical derived from some mushrooms) and nicotine well before they knew about acetylcholine. Muscarinic receptors bind muscarine, and nicotinic receptors bind nicotine. After they were discovered and researched, acetylcholine was discovered and determined to bind with both muscarinic and nicotinic receptors; but by then many publications had been printed over the years and it was easier to keep the "muscarinic" and "nicotinic" names than to start over.

Acetylcholine binds with at least seven known different types of receptors. Acetylcholine binds with muscarinic receptors, which are labeled: M_1, M_2, M_3, M_4, and M_5. It also binds with nicotinic receptors, which are labeled N_n and N_m, the small "n" stands for "neuronal" and the small "m" stands for "muscle."

Muscarinic receptors are located in sweat glands, the CNS, autonomic ganglia, the heart, smooth muscle (bladder), and secretory glands. Muscarinic receptors are a subset of G protein-coupled receptors. Muscarinic receptors initiate biochemical cascades. In the heart, these cascades decrease heart rate. In contrast, in the lungs, these cascades increase bronchial secretions.

Nicotinic receptors are located at the neuromuscular junction, autonomic ganglia, adrenal medulla, and neurons in the central nervous system. Nicotinic receptors are ligand-gated ion channels. This means their activation allows sodium ions to enter cells when the receptor is stimulated by agonists. This leads to conduction of nerve impulses or skeletal muscle contraction.

CHOLINERGIC DRUGS

Cholinergic drugs mimic acetylcholine's effects. Cholinergic drugs divide into two classes: 1) direct acting - drugs binding directly with muscarinic and/or nicotinic receptors, or 2) indirect acting - drugs prolonging acetylcholine's half-life by inhibiting acetylcholinesterase.

Cholinergic drugs treat Alzheimer's Disease, myasthenia gravis, glaucoma, urinary retention, paralytic ileus, head lice, reverse life-threatening effects of anticholinergic overdoses, dry-mouth, cause miosis for cataract surgery, reverse the effects of non-depolarizing neuromuscular blocking drugs, and help diagnose hyperreactive bronchial airway disease.

DIRECT ACTING AGONISTS

The direct acting cholinomimetic drugs include acetylcholine, bethanechol, carbachol, methacholine, pilocarpine, nicotine, and varenicline. Acetylcholine, bethanechol, carbachol, and methacholine are all choline esters, just as acetylcholine is a choline ester. Pilocarpine is an alkaloid, structurally similar to muscarine.

Acetylcholine causes beneficial miosis during various eye surgeries, including cataract surgery. A dose of 0.5 ml to 2 ml, injected into the anterior chamber of the eye, produces miosis for about ten minutes. Because of its parasympathetic effects, acetylcholine may cause difficulty breathing, hypotension, and bradycardia.

Bethanechol, structurally similar to acetylcholine and approved for urinary retention, increases the bladder's contractile force during urination. It also treats postoperative gastrointestinal atony and gastric retention. Bethanechol preferentially binds with muscarinic receptors over nicotinic receptors. Bethanechol causes the same side-effects as acetylcholine.

Carbachol, approved for glaucoma, lowers pressure within the eye. Carbachol is not administered orally because of severe toxicity; systemic absorption from opthalmic administration is minimal. Methacholine is used to diagnose bronchial airway disease by stimulating an airway response.

Varenicline helps people quit smoking. As an agonist at the alpha-4 beta-2 nicotinic acetylcholine receptor, patients experience less withdrawal symptoms than quitting cold turkey. Further, patients experience less psychological craving for tobacco products. It can cause headaches, abnormal dreams, and insomnia.

INDIRECT ACTING AGONISTS

The indirect acting cholinomimetics include neostigmine, physostigmine, pyridostigmine, malathion, and edrophonium. These drugs all inhibit the enzyme acetylcholinesterase, which is responsible for metabolizing acetylcholine. Inhibiting acetylcholinesterase increases the amount of time that each acetylcholine molecule lasts in the synapse between neurons, thus increasing the amount of acetylcholine in a synapse. Neostigmine, physostigmine, and pyridostigmine are carbamic esters of choline. Their chemical structures allow them to bind with acetylcholinesterase for hours; thus effectively increasing the half-life of acetylcholine from seconds to hours.

Neostigmine and pyridostigmine treat myasthenia gravis and, after surgery, reverse the effects of non-depolarizing neuromuscular blockers. Myasthenia gravis is characterized by auto-antibodies binding with nicotinic acetylcholine receptors at the neuromuscular junction, resulting in less receptors available for acetylcholine to bind with. Without acetylcholine binding at these receptors, patients experience marked physical weakness.

Pyridostigmine is also used as prophylaxis for exposure to soman, a chemical warfare agent ("nerve gas"); it must be administered well before exposure to be effective.

Physostigmine treats glaucoma and atropine overdoses. Physostigmine, being a tertiary amine, lacks the positive charge the quaternary amines have, allowing entry into the CNS to treat poisoning from anticholinergic agents.

Edrophonium is used to diagnose myasthenia gravis and reverse blockade of nicotinic receptors at the neuromuscular end-plate. It lasts for about 5 to 10 minutes. Edrophonium is the only marketed acetylcholinesterase inhibitor that has an alcohol structure and lacks an ester structure. As a quaternary amine, it poorly penetrates the CNS.

Echothiophate, an organophosphate ester, treats open angle glaucoma. It is dosed twice daily. Its severe potency when administered systemically limits its use to opthalmic applications.

Malathion, also an organophosphate ester, treats scabies. As an organophosphate ester, its chemical structure allows it to bind essentially irreversibly with acetylcholinesterase. After systemic exposure, it takes days to weeks to recover. As a topical drug, malathion treats scabies, but does not have any internal therapeutic uses in humans. Organophosphate esters were originally developed as insecticides in the early 1900's, and upon realization of their harm to humans, were turned into chemical warfare agents (nerve gas, sarin, etc.). Organophosphate esters are considered to be irreversible inhibitors of acetylcholinesterase.

ACETYLCHOLINESTERASE INHIBITORS FOR ALZHEIMER'S DISEASE

Acetylcholine is vitally important to cognitive functioning, and influences cognitive function in patients with Alzheimer's Disease. Rivastigmine, galantamine, and donepezil all inhibit acetylcholinesterase, thus increasing acetylcholine levels in the brain. For some patients, these drugs alter their scores on cognitive exams; however, none have been shown to alter the course of Alzheimer's Disease.

SIDE-EFFECTS

Cholinomimetic drugs cause a range of side-effects, including: salivation, lacrimation, urination, defecation, upset GI tract, vomiting, pupil constriction, and muscle spasms. When resulting from therapeutic doses of pharmacologic drugs, these side-effects are usually self-limiting. When resulting from exposure to insecticides or chemical warfare agents, patients will need emergency treatment consisting of atropine and pralidoxime, along with airway and cardiac support.

DRUG INTERACTIONS

Overall, cholinomimetic drugs do not interfere with hepatic CYP450 isoenzymes. Further, they do not cause plasma protein-binding interactions. Their interactions include additive effects occurring when they are administered with other drugs causing cholinergic effects.

ANTICHOLINERGIC DRUGS

Anticholinergic drugs can be classified as either antimuscarinic or antinicotinic drugs. Antinicotinic drugs are further divided into ganglion blockers and neuromuscular blockers. Ganglion blockers were once used, but have been replaced by newer medications having fewer adverse effects.

ANTIMUSCARINIC DRUGS

Muscarinic receptor antagonists treat a variety of medical conditions including: motion sickness, Parkinson's disease, urinary urgency problems, chronic obstructive pulmonary disease, acute use for cardiac conditions, and opthalmic conditions. This reflects the diversity of biological processes influenced by acetylcholine. Most antimuscarinic drugs are relatively non-selective for the receptors they bind with, thus causing unwanted off-target side-effects.

Antimuscarinic drugs include atropine, benztropine, dicyclomine, flavoxate, glycopyrrolate, homatropine, oxybutynin, scopolamine, tolterodine, and trihexyphenidyl. Antimuscarinic drugs all inhibit acetylcholine at muscarinic receptors.

Atropine, an alkaloid, inhibits acetylcholine at muscarinic receptors. Atropine has a panoply of therapeutic benefits ranging from dilating the eyes for opthalmologic exams, preanesthetic to stop salivation and lung secretions, reversing symptomatic sinus bradycardia, and antidote for acetylcholinesterase inhibitor poisoning, and reduces side-effects of acetylcholinesterase inhibitors, which are used for reversal of neuromuscular blockade. Homatropine, like atropine, causes mydriasis and cycloplegia (inability to focus the eye muscles), necessary conditions for some opthalmic exams and procedures.

Atropine, at normal doses, does not appreciably cross the blood-brain barrier. However, at toxic doses, atropine readily crosses the blood-brain barrier, causing serious adverse effects. The liver metabolizes atropine, but it does not have any consequential drug-drug interactions; and it does not displace other drugs from plasma-proteins. It has a half-life of two hours. The effects of atropine eye drops can last for 24 hours to 72 hours.

Antimuscarinic drugs are commonly used to treat overactive bladder problems. Acetylcholine causes bladder contractions; antagonism of acetylcholine at muscarinic receptors in the bladder relieves overactive bladder for some patients. Antimuscarinic drugs that treat overactive bladder include flavoxate, solifenacin, tolterodine, trospium, fesoterodine, darifenacin, and oxybutynin. These drugs treat overactive bladder by competitively antagonizing the effects of acetylcholine on the bladder. They are all generally equally effective; however, individual patients may prefer one in particular. Dry mouth (xerostomia) is a common side-effect of these medications.

Scopolamine treats motion sickness by blocking muscarinic receptors in the central nervous system. Scopolamine, as a tertiary amine, readily crosses the blood-brain barrier. It is administered as a patch that lasts for three days. Anticholinergic drugs for respiratory problems and Parkinson's disease are discussed in their respective chapters.

SIDE-EFFECTS

Atropine, like all anticholinergics, can cause severe dry mouth, ataxia (loss of physical coordination), hyperthermia from decreased sweating, pupil dilation, cycloplegia (blurred vision), diplopia (double vision), tachycardia (increased heart rate), urinary retention, constipation, and increased intraocular pressure. Central nervous system side-effects of atropine include agitation, sedation, dizziness, disorientation, euphoria, dysphoria, incoherent speech, seizures, visual disturbances, coma, and death. Acetylcholinesterase inhibitors can antagonize the toxic effects of atropine.

ANTINICOTINIC NEUROMUSCULAR BLOCKERS

Neuromuscular blockers can be divided into depolarizing and non-depolarizing drugs. Both classes cause paralysis during surgery.

Depolarizing neuromuscular blockers are initially agonists at the acetylcholine nicotinic-receptor in skeletal muscle; however, after initial depolarization, they stay bound to the receptor, thus causing persistent depolarization, so, in effect, they block the next neuronal release of acetylcholine from causing muscle contraction, in that regard, they are considered antagonists. Succinylcholine is the only depolarizing neuromuscular blocker available in the U.S.

Non-depolarizing neuromuscular blockers are antagonists at the acetylcholine nicotinic-receptor in skeletal muscle. They paralyze skeletal muscle. Tubocurarine is probably the most well known member of this group (these are the arrow poisons originating from South America). Other members include atracurium, pancuronium, and vecuronium.

GANGLIONIC BLOCKERS

Much earlier, several ganglionic blockers were clinically used, but today drugs with more receptor specificity, and, hence, less side-effects, are used.

Direct Acting Cholinergic Drugs				
Generic Name / Brand Name	Clinical Use	Dose	Dosage Form	Mechanism of Action
Acetylcholine Miochol®-E	Causes rapid miosis for cataract surgery and other eye surgeries	Adult: 0.5-2 ml of 1% solution	Miochol®-E 20 mg/2ml vial	Agonist at the M_3 receptor causing pupil constriction (miosis)
Bethanechol Urecholine®	Urinary retention and neurogenic bladder	Adult initial dose: 10-50 mg 3 to 4 times daily, max dose of 400 mg per 24 hours	Tablets: 5, 10, 25, 50 mg	Increases bladder muscle contractile force, thus de-creasing urinary retention
Carbachol Miostat® Isopto®-Car-bachol	Glaucoma Causes miosis for surgery	Adult glaucoma dose: instill 1-2 drops three times daily. Miosis for surgery: Instill 0.5 ml into anterior chamber be-fore or after securing sutures	Isopto® Carbachol Ophthalmic solution: 1.5% 15 ml; 3% 15 ml Miostat® 0.01% 1.5 ml bottle	Agonist at the M_3 receptor causing miosis, allowing fluid to drain from the eye, thus decreasing pressure
Methacholine Provocholine®	Diagnosis of bronchial airway hyperreactivity	Adults and children 5 years and older: 5 breaths of successive strengths starting at 0.025 mg/ml and increasing to 0.25 etc. See manufacturer's detailed instructions in package insert	Powder for reconstitu-tion: 100 mg per vial	Patients who have bronchial hyper-reactivity will produce excessive bronchial secre-tions
Pilocarpine Isopto®-Carpine, Salagen®	Salagen®: dry mouth re-sulting from decreased salivary gland function caused by radiotherapy for cancer of head and neck. Isopto-Carpine®: open-angle glaucoma, acute angle-closure glaucoma, induction of miosis	Adult initial dose for xerostomia: 5 mg three times daily, may increase to 10 mg TID Adult glaucoma dose: 1-2 drops upto 6 times daily	Salagen® tablets 5 and 7.5 mg Isopto® Carpine 1% 15ml, 2% 15ml, 4% 15ml	Stimulates sal-ivary glands to produce saliva; Treats glaucoma by causing miosis, thus allowing flu-id to drain from the eye

Direct Acting Cholinergic Drugs

Generic Name / Brand Name	Clinical Use	Dose	Dosage Form	Mechanism of Action
Nicotine Nicotrol Inhaler®	Smoking cessation	Inhale contents of 6 to 16 cartridges daily spaced every 20 minutes; taper initial dose after 6 to 12 weeks. Quit smoking when starting treatment.	Nicotrol® Inhaler 10 mg per inhaler	Replaces nicotine from cigarettes, allowing for gradual reduction of dose, lessening withdrawal symptoms
Varenicline Chantix®	Smoking cessation	Starting month box: 0.5 mg once daily for 3 days, then 0.5 mg twice daily for 4 days, then 1 mg twice daily; quit smoking within 8 to 35 days of starting drug	Starting month box is titrated. Maintenance box have 56 1 mg tablets.	Partial agonist at alpha-4-beta-2 nicotinic acetylcholine receptor, decreasing cravings and withdrawal symptoms

Acetylcholinesterase Inhibitors: Indirect Acting Cholinergic Drugs

Generic Name / Brand Name	Clinical Use	Dose	Dosage Form	Mechanism of Action / Half-life / Duration of action
Chemical class: Carbamates				
Neostigmine Prostigmin®	Myasthenia gravis, reversal of non-depolarizing neuromuscular blocking drugs, paralytic ileus, urinary retention	Treat myasthenia gravis: usual adult starting dose: 15 mg 3 times daily; maintenance dose range: 15 mg to 375 mg daily in divided doses every 3 to 4 hours. Adult dose, reversal of non-depolarizing neuromuscular blockade: IV 0.5-2 mg prn, max total dose of 5 mg;	Prostigmin® tablet 15 mg; Injection solution: 0.5 mg/ml 10 ml vial, 1 mg/ml 10 ml vial	Reversibly inhibits acetylcholinesterase. Half-life: 1 hour. Duration of action: IM 2.5 to 4 hours; IV 1 to 2 hours
Physostigmine	Reverses overdose of anticholinergics	Adult dose: IM or IV 0.5-2 mg initially, dose every 10-30 minutes prn	Solution for injection: 1 mg/ml 2 ml vials	Same as above. Half-life: 15 to 40 minutes. Duration: 1 to 2 hours

Acetylcholinesterase Inhibitors: Indirect Acting Cholinergic Drugs

Generic Name / Brand Name	Clinical Use	Dose	Dosage Form	Mechanism of Action / Half-life / Duration of action
Pyridostigmine Bromide Mestinon® Regonol®	Mestinon® : Myasthenia gravis Regonol®: reversal of nondepolarizing neuromuscular blockers.	Treat myasthenia gravis: usual adult starting dose: 60 mg three times daily; maintenance dose range: 60 mg to 1500 mg daily in divided doses Adult dose reversal of non-depolarizing neuromuscular blockers: 0.1-0.25 mg/kg/dose	Generic tablets 60 mg; Mestinon® tablets 60 mg immediate release and 180 mg extended release; Regonol® solution for injection: 5 mg/ml 2 ml	Same as above. Half-life: 1 to 2 hours for IV and 3 hours orally. Duration of action: IV 2 to 3 hours; orally 6 to 8 hours

Chemical class: Organophosphorus (Organophosphates)

Echothiophate Iodide Phospholine Iodide®	Chronic open angle glaucoma	Adult dose: usually 1 drop twice daily	Phospholine Iodide® 6.25 mg/5ml	Irreversibly binds to acetylcholinesterase
Malathion Ovide®	Head lice	Adults and children 6 and over: thoroughly apply to dry hair and scalp, rinse after 8-12 hours, repeat in 7-9 days if needed	Ovide® topical lotion 0.5% 59ml; generic 0.5% 59 ml	Same as above.

Chemical class: Alcohol

Edrophonium Enlon®	Diagnose myasthenia gravis; Reversal of non-depolarizing neuromuscular blockade	Adult dose reversal of non-depolarizing neuromuscular blocker: IV 10 mg, repeat if needed every 5 to 10 minutes, max of 40 mg total dose	Enlon® injection solution 10 mg/ml 15 ml vial	Reversibly inhibits acetylcholinesterase. Half-life: 1.2 to 2.4 hours. Duration of action; IM 5 to 30 minutes; IV 10 minutes

Muscarinic Antagonists

Generic Name / Brand Name	Clinical Use	Dose	Dosage Form	Mechanism of Action
Atropine Isopto® Atropine	Induce mydriasis for ophthalmic examinations, symptomatic sinus bradycardia, inhibit salivation and mucus production during surgery, cholinergic poisoning, chemical warfare agent poisoning	Mydriasis: 1 to 2 drops in eye(s) Bradycardia: 0.5 mg IV every 3 to 5 minutes as needed Organophosphate / insecticide poisoning: 1 to 2 mg IM or IV every 10 minutes as needed	Isopto® Atropine 1% solution Various strengths of pre-filled syringes and vials: 1mg/ml; 0.8 mg/ ml	Blocks muscarinic receptors in the eye, preventing acetylcholine from binding with muscarinic receptors

Muscarinic Antagonists				
Generic Name / Brand Name	Clinical Use	Dose	Dosage Form	Mechanism of Action
Benztropine Cogentin®	Parkinson's Disease	Drug induced extrapyramidal symptoms: 1-4 mg one to two times daily	Tablets 0.5 mg, 1 mg, and 2 mg; Solution for injection 1 mg/ml	Antagonist at muscarinic receptors
Dicyclomine Bentyl®	Irritable bowel syndrome	Adult oral initial dose: 20 mg four times daily, may increase to 40 mg four times daily if needed	Tablet and capsules 20 mg	Inhibits M_2 receptors, preventing acetylcholine from binding, thus slowing GI motility
Flavoxate Urispas®	Spasms in bladder	Adults and children older than 12: 100-200 mg orally 3 to 4 times daily	Tablet 100 mg	Inhibits muscarinic receptors, preventing acetylcholine from binding
Glycopyrrolate Robinul®, Robinul® Forte	Reduces salivary, tracheobronchial, and pharyngeal secretions preoperatively. For peptic ulcer when oral medication cannot be used.	Adult reduction of secretions, preoperative IM dose: 4 mcg/kg 30-60 minutes before surgery	Solution for injection: 0.2 mg/ml 1, 2, 5, and 20 ml vials	Inhibits muscarinic receptors, preventing the binding of acetylcholine, which would increase secretions
Homatropine Isopto® Homatropine	Causes cycloplegia and mydriasis for refraction	Adult dose: 2% solution 1-2 drops just before procedure, 5% solution 1 drop before procedure	Isopto® Homatropine 2% and 5% 5 ml each	Inhibits muscarinic receptors, preventing acetylcholine from binding
Oxybutynin Ditropan®, Gelnique®, Oxytrol®	Urgency, frequency, leakage, urge incontinence, and dysuria	Adult dose: 5 mg 2 to 3 times daily	Tablet: 5 mg; Ditropan® Extended Release tablets: 5, 10, 15 mg; Syrup: 5 mg/5ml 473 ml; Oxytrol® patch: 3.9 mg/24 hours; Gelnique gel®: 10%	Blocks muscarinic receptors, particularly in the CNS; as a tertiary amine, it readily enters the CNS
Scopolamine Transderm Scop®	The patch treats motion sickness.	One patch applied to skin every 3 days.	Patch 1.5 mg.	Blocks muscarinic receptors, particularly in the CNS; as a tertiary amine, it readily enters the CNS

Page 30

Muscarinic Antagonists				
Generic Name / Brand Name	Clinical Use	Dose	Dosage Form	Mechanism of Action
Tolterodine Detrol®	Overactive bladder with symptoms of urge urinary incontinence, urgency, and frequency.	2 mg BID; extended release capsules: 2-4 mg once daily	Detrol® tablets: 1 and 2 mg; Detrol® LA extended release capsules: 2 and 4 mg	Competitively inhibits muscarinic receptors, thus decreasing detrusor muscle pressure
Trihexyphenidyl Artane®	Drug-induced extrapyramidal symptoms; Parkinson's Disease	Initial EPS dose: 1 mg once daily, maintenance dose: 5 mg once to three times daily: Parkinson's Disease initial dose: 1 mg once daily, maintenance dose: 6-10 mg a day split into 3 doses	Tablets: 2 and 5 mg	Inhibits acetylcholine receptors in the CNS to realign the balance between acetylcholine and dopamine, which work together to control muscular movements

CHAPTER 4

SYMPATHOMIMETICS AND SYM-PATHOLYTIC DRUGS

Sympathomimetic Agonists		Sympatholytics	
Direct acting	Indirect Acting	Alpha Blockers	Beta Blockers
Epinephrine Norepinephrine Dopamine Dobutamine Albuterol Phenylephrine	Cause release of neurotransmitter and block its reuptake: Amphetamines Monoamine Oxidase Inhibitors (MAOI): Selegiline Isocarboxazid Phenelzine Tranylcypromine	Selective: Prazosin Terazosin Doxazosin Non-Selective: Phenoxybenzamine Phentolamine	Selective: Atenolol Metoprolol Non-Selective: Propranolol Labetalol

Direct acting sympathomimetic drugs treat many medical conditions including asthma (albuterol); cardiac arrest and anaphylactic shock (epinephrine); shock and severe hypotension (norepinephrine); myocardial infarction, renal failure, or cardiac decompensation (dopamine); short-term treatment of cardiac decompensation (dobutamine); and stuffy nose and vasoconstrictor for local analgesia (phenylephrine).

Indirect acting sympathomimetics treat depression (MAOI), attention deficit disorder (amphetamines), and Parkinson's disease (MAOI).

Excessively high blood pressure or increased heart rate are side-effects of sympathomimetic agonists. Monoamine oxidase inhibitors cause hypertension when taken with some red wines and some cheeses.

Sympatholytics treat high blood pressure by various mechanisms. Beta-blockers decrease the heart's contractile force. Alpha-blockers prevent norepinephrine from constricting arteries and veins, thus decreasing blood pressure, sometimes too much. Alpha blockers are known for decreasing blood pressure so much that some people faint, particularly the elderly. Advise patients to take them just before bed to reduce the risk of falls.

Beta-blockers can decrease heart rate excessively, cause heart block, and cause breathing problems. Further diabetic patients should be warned that beta-blockers can mask the signs of hypoglycemia.

Sympathomimetic agonists are either direct acting or indirect acting. Direct acting drugs bind directly with alpha and/or beta receptors. Indirect acting drugs increase the amount of neurotransmitter in the synapse by either increasing the release of neurotransmitters or blocking the reuptake of neurotransmitters. Ultimately, this increases the actions of norepinephrine, epinephrine, and/or dopamine.

DIRECT ACTING

Direct-acting sympathomimetic drugs work by directly binding with alpha, beta, and/or dopamine receptors. Sympathomimetic drugs treat anaphylaxis, shock, heart failure, nasal congestion, red eyes, asthma, and other conditions.

Commonly used direct-acting sympathomimetics include epinephrine (anaphylactic shock and cardiac arrest), norepinephrine (shock and severe hypotension), dopamine (myocardial infarction, renal failure, or cardiac decompensation), dobutamine (short-term treatment of cardiac decompensation), albuterol (asthma), and phenylephrine (stuffy nose, vasoconstrictor for local analgesia).

In general, most direct-acting sympathomimetics bind with several different sympathomimetic receptors. This is because of the close similarity in drug structures and close similarity in receptor structures. Epinephrine, for example, binds with both alpha receptors and all three beta receptors. Norepinephrine, in contrast, binds with both alpha receptors and just the beta-1 receptor. Dopamine, at high enough doses, binds with not only the dopamine-1 receptor (D_1), but also both alpha receptors and all three beta receptors.

Albuterol preferentially binds with $beta_2$ receptors, causing bronchodilation. Albuterol can cause tachycardia (abnormally fast heart rate) in some patients by binding with $beta_2$ receptors in the heart. The heart has both $beta_1$ and $beta_2$ receptors. Phenylephrine, in contrast to albuterol, binds with alpha receptors, but not with beta receptors.

INDIRECT ACTING

Indirect-acting sympathomimetics cross the blood-brain barrier where they are used to treat attention-deficit disorders, depression, and Parkinson's disease. Their chemical structures prevent MAO from metabolizing them.

Indirect-acting sympathomimetics have three main mechanisms of action: 1) blocking the reuptake of neurotransmitters back into the releasing neuron, 2) stimulating neurons to release neurotransmitters, and 3) slowing the metabolism of neurotransmitters.

Amphetamines and their derivatives are believed to cause neurons to both release norepinephrine and dopamine into synapses and block the reuptake of these neurotransmitters back into the neuron that released them. An increase in norepinephrine and/or dopamine treats some forms of depression and attention-deficit hyperactivity disorders.

Monoamine oxidase inhibitors (MAOIs) include selegiline, isocarboxazid, phenelzine, and tranylcypromine. They prevent the metabolism of norepinephrine and dopamine (and serotonin, but serotonin is not a sympathomimetic neurotransmitter). MAOIs treat depression and/or Parkinson's disease. Care must be taken not to administer MAOIs with red wine or some cheeses because they contain tyramine (a monoamine), which can substantially raise blood-pressure. MAOIs prevent the metabolism of tyramine.

SYMPATHOLYTICS

Sympatholytic drugs are used to treat cardiovascular problems, such as, high blood pressure (hypertension), excessive heart rate (tachycardia), and myocardial infarction.

BETA-BLOCKERS

Beta-blockers are traditionally divided into non-selective and selective beta-blockers. Non-selective beta-blockers block both $beta_1$ and $beta_2$ receptors. Selective beta-blockers block $beta_1$ receptors. Activation of $beta_2$ receptors keeps the lungs open, making it easier to breathe; blocking $beta_2$ receptors causes serious breathing problems, leading to death in some patients. Initially, non-selective beta-blockers were discovered; later $beta_1$ selective blockers were discovered.

Today, atenolol and metoprolol are the main selective $beta_1$ blockers used to treat high blood pressure, tachycardia, or myocardial infarction (after the patient has stabilized). They are inexpensive and work well.

Propranolol, a non-selective beta-blocker, is a tertiary treatment for migraine headaches and panic attacks. Timolol, a non-selective beta-blocker treats glaucoma. It is available in several different opthalmic preparations (short-acting and long-acting).

Interestingly, carvedilol and labetalol each block both beta receptors and $alpha_1$ receptors. Carvedilol is indicated to treat mild to severe chronic heart failure, left ventricular dysfunction after myocardial infarction in clinically stable patients, and hypertension. Labetalol is indicated to treat hypertension. It is especially effective with loop or thiazide diuretics.

Beta blockers are commonly used with other anti-hypertensive drugs. The combination of two antihypertensive drugs may result in severe hypotension. When combining two drugs, start with the lowest possible dose of the second drug to reduce the possibility of severe hypotension.

ALPHA- BLOCKERS

Older, non-selective alpha blockers, such as, phenoxybenzamine and phentolamine, compete with norepinephrine and epinephrine for binding with $alpha_1$ and $alpha_2$ receptors located in both arterioles and veins. Blocking alpha receptors in arteries and veins dilates them, thus lowering blood pressure. The blocking of $alpha_2$ receptors causes unwanted side-effects such as postural hypotension and reflex tachycardia, which may cause heart arrhythmias. Consequently, phenoxybenzamine and phentolamine generally are not the first choice for treating hypertension. However, phenoxybenzamine and phentolamine are used to treat patients with pheochromocytoma.

Prazosin, terazosin, and doxazosin are selective

alpha$_1$ receptor blockers used for hypertension. All should be initially administered at bedtime because of possible postural hypotension, which may cause a patient to fall.

In addition to treating hypertension, terazosin and doxazosin also treat benign prostatic hypertrophy (BPH). BPH is the enlargement of the prostate gland. Enlargement of this gland usually causes urinary prob-lems. Some experience difficulty completely emptying their bladder and may experience frequent urination as a result. Both, block alpha$_1$ receptors, causing the smooth muscle around the bladder opening to relax, al-lowing unobstructed urination, and allowing complete emptying of the bladder.

Direct Acting Sympathomimetics				
Generic Name / Brand Name	Indication	Dose	Dosage Form	Mechanism of Action
Epinephrine Adrenalin®	Asystole	Adult dose asystole/ pulseless arrest: IV 1 mg every 3 to 5 minutes until return of circulation	Injection: 1 mg/ml 30 ml vial	Stimulates both alpha receptors and all three beta receptors
Dobutamine	Short-term treatment of cardiac decompen-sation	Adult and child dose: IV 2 mcg-20 mcg/ kg/min IV, max of 40 mcg/kg/min	Injection solution: 12.5 mg/ml in 20 and 40 ml vials; Premixed in D$_5$W as 1 mg/ml in 250 ml bags	Stimulates beta$_1$ receptors increasing heart rate and heart contractility, slight effect on beta$_2$ and alpha receptors
Dopamine	Shock	Adult dose: IV 1-50 mcg/kg/min	Injection solution: 40 mg/ml in 5 and 10 ml vials; 80 mg/ml in 5 ml vials; 160 mg/ml in 5 ml vials	Low doses dilate vessels thus lower-ing cardiac work-load in patients with heart failure; High doses stimulate alpha receptors thus increasing blood pressure in patients experiencing shock
Isoproterenol Isuprel®	Mild and transient episodes of heart block; shock	Adult dose for shock: 0.5 mcg to 5 mcg per minute.	Injection: Isuprel® 0.2 mg/ml, 1 and 5 ml vials	Stimulates beta$_1$ and beta$_2$ receptors, increasing heart rate and contractility
Norepinephrine Levophed®	Treatment of shock, severe hypotension	Adult dose: IV 2-12 mcg/min	Injection: 1 mg/ml 4 ml vial	Stimulates both alpha receptors and beta$_1$

Centrally Acting Alpha-2 Agonists Sympathomimetics

Generic Name / Brand Name	Use	Dose	Dosage Form	Mechanism of Action
Clonidine Catapres®	Hypertension	Adult initial dose: 0.1 mg twice daily; maintenance dose 0.2 mg to 0.6 mg per day in divided doses.	Tablets: 0.1 mg, 0.2 mg, and 0.3 mg	In the CNS, as an agonist at alpha$_2$ receptors, it causes the CNS to decrease sympathetic outflow to the periphery, thus decreasing blood pressure
Guanabenz Wytensin	Hypertension	Initial adult dose 4 mg to 8 mg BID, maintenance dose: titrate as needed every 1 to 2 weeks, max dose of 32 mg twice daily	Tablet 4 mg	Same as above
Guanfacine Intuniv® Tenex®	Tenex treats hypertension. Intuniv treats Attention deficit disorder, Attention deficit hyperactivity disorder	Adult dose Tenex®: 1 mg at bedtime, maintenance dose: 0.5-2 mg at bedtime	Tenex® tablets 1 and 2 mg; Intuniv® tablets 1, 2, 3, and 4 mg	Same as above
Methyldopa Aldomet®	Hypertension	Adult initial oral dose: 250 mg two to three times daily in first 48 hours, then increase or decrease dose every 2 days. Usual daily dose is 500 mg to 2 g in 2 to 4 doses.	Tablets 250 and 500 mg; Injection solution 50 mg/ml	Same as above
Reserpine	Mild to moderate hypertension	Adult initial dose: 0.1 mg once daily, adult maintenance dose: 0.05-0.25 mg once daily	Tablets: 0.1 and 0.25 mg	In central and peripheral adrenergic neurons, reserpine prevents storage vesicles from storing neurotransmitters such as dopamine and norepinephrine, this causes dopamine and norepinephrine to leak into the synaptic junction and be metabolized, resulting in a loss of sympathetic stimulation, causing decreased blood pressure

Non-Selective Alpha Blockers

Generic Name / Brand Name	Use	Dose	Dosage Form	Mechanism of Action
Phenoxybenzamine Dibenzyline®	Pheochromocytoma	Initially 10 mg twice daily. Increase dose every other day to the range of 20 mg to 40 mg 2 to 3 times daily.	Dibenzyline® capsule 10 mg	Blocks both alpha receptors

Phentolamine OraVerse®	Pheochromocy-toma	5 mg IV or IM every 1 to 2 hours as needed before oper-ation.	Injection solu-tion: 5 mg vials; Oraverse dental cartridge 0.4 mg/1.7 ml	Same as above

Selective Alpha$_1$ Blockers Relative to Alpha$_2$

Doxazosin Cardura® Cardura® XL	Benign prostatic hypertrophy, hypertension	Initial dose for BPH or hyper-tension 1 mg once daily in the morning or evening. Postural hypotension occurs 2 to 6 hours after dose. BPH mainte-nance dose: 1 mg to 8 mg QD. Hypertension 1 mg to 16 mg QD.	Tablets imme-diate release: 1, 2, 4, and 8 mg; Extended release tablets 4 and 8 mg	Blocks alpha$_{1A}$, al-pha$_{1B}$, and alpha$_{1D}$ receptors
Prazosin Minipress®	Hypertension	Initial dose: 1 mg two to three times daily. Usual range 6 mg to 15 mg in divided doses. Dose higher than 20 mg are usually not beneficial, however some patient respond at 40 mg in divided doses.	Capsules 1 mg, 2 mg, and 5 mg	Blocks alpha$_{1A}$, al-pha$_{1B}$, and alpha$_{1D}$ receptors
Terazosin Hytrin®	Benign prostat-ic hyperplasia, hypertension	Initial dose for BPH and hypertension: 1 mg orally at bedtime. Most patients stay within 1 mg to 5 mg QD. Some patients may need 20 mg QD.	Capsules: 1 mg, 2 mg, 5 mg, and 10 mg	Blocks alpha$_{1A}$, al-pha1$_B$, and alpha$_{1D}$ receptors
Alfuzosin Uroxatral®	Benign prostatic hyperplasia	Adult dose: 10 mg once daily	Tablet extended release: 10 mg	Blocks alpha$_{1A}$, al-pha$_{1B}$, and alpha$_{1D}$ receptors
Tamsulosin Flomax®	Benign prostatic hyperplasia	0.4 mg once daily, 30 minutes after the same meal each day. May increase to 0.8 mg once daily after 2-4 weeks if lower dose does not work.	Capsule: 0.4 mg	Selectively blocks alpha$_{1A}$ and alpha$_{1D}$ receptors relative to alpha$_{1B}$
Silodosin Rapaflo®	Benign prostatic hyperplasia	8 mg PO QD with food. 4 mg PO QD for patients with moderate renal impairment, creatine clearance 30-50 ml/min.	Capsules: 4 mg and 8 mg	Selectively blocks alpha$_{1A}$

Indirect Sympathomimetics: Increasing Norepinephrine release and blocking reuptake

Generic Name / Brand Name	Use	Dose	Dosage Form	Mechanism of Ac-tion
Dextroamphet-amine Adderall XR®	Attention deficit disorder, Attention deficit hyperactivity disorder	Adult and child dose: 5-30mg once daily in the morning	Capsules: 5, 10, 15, 20, 25, 30 mg	Causes presynaptic neurons to release dopamine and norepinephrine and block reuptake

Indirect Sympathomimetics: Increasing Norepinephrine release and blocking reuptake				
Generic Name / Brand Name	Use	Dose	Dosage Form	Mechanism of Action
Methamphet-amine Desoxyn®	Attention deficit disorder, Attention deficit hyperactivity disorder	Adult and children older than 6 start at 5 mg once to twice daily. May increase if needed to 25 mg daily in divided doses. Increase daily dose by 5 mg once weekly	Tablet 5 mg	Same as above
Methylphenidate Concerta® Methylin® Ritalin®	Attention deficit disorder, Attention deficit hyperactivity disorder	Children ages 6 to 12: initial dose of 18 mg daily; if needed may increase to 36 mg daily after one week; Maximum dose of 2 mg/kg/day upto 54 mg. Adult dose: Concerta® 18-54 mg once daily in the morning; increase by 18 mg once weekly if needed	Concerta® tablets: 18, 27, 36, 54 mg	Blocks presynaptic neurons from reuptaking norepinephrine and dopamine

CHAPTER 5

ANTIDEPRESSANTS

Monoamine Oxidase Inhibitors	Tricyclic Antidepressants	Selective Serotonin Reuptake Inhibitors	Serotonin-Norepi-nephrine Reuptake Inhibitors	Atypical Antidepressants
Isocarboxazid Phenelzine Tranylcypromine	Amitriptyline Clomipramine Doxepin Imipramine Amoxapine Desipramine Maprotiline Nortriptyline Protriptyline	Citalopram Escitalopram Fluoxetine Fluvoxamine Paroxetine Sertraline	Desvenlafaxine Duloxetine Milnacipran Venlafaxine	Bupropion Mirtazapine Trazodone

Most antidepressants treat depression by raising levels of serotonin and norepinephrine. Monoamine oxidase inhibitors prevent the enzyme monoamine oxidase from metabolizing norepinephrine and serotonin, thus increasing the amount of these neurotransmitters in the brain. Tricyclic antidepressants work by preventing presynaptic neurons from reuptaking norepinephrine and serotonin back into the nerve terminal. Selective serotonin reuptake inhibitors (SSRIs) work by competitively blocking serotonin transporters in presynaptic neurons from reuptaking serotonin back into the nerve terminal. This leaves serotonin in the synapse for a longer time, decreasing depression symptoms. Serotonin-Norepinephrine Reuptake Inhibitors (SNRIs) prevent transporters from reuptaking serotonin and norepinephrine back into presynaptic neurons, thus leaving serotonin and norepinephrine in the synapse for a longer time, decreasing depression symptoms. Bupropion, an atypical antidepressant, weakly inhibits the reuptake of dopamine and norepinephrine back into presynaptic neurons. Mirtazapine is an antagonist at central presynaptic alpha$_2$ adrenergic inhibitory auto-receptors and hetero-receptors; this is believed to increase the activity of serotonin and norepinephrine in the brain. Trazodone selectively inhibits neuronal reuptake of serotonin and is an antagonist at 5-HT$_{2A/2C}$ serotonin receptors.

MAOIs can cause severe hypertension when coadministered with some sympathomimetic drugs because MAOIs prevent the metabolism of some sympathomimetic drugs. Further MAOIs can cause severe hypertension when coadministered with red wine and some cheeses. Red wine and some cheeses have tyramine (tyramine is a monoamine); tyramine can substantially raise blood pressure.

SSRIs and SNRIs can cause "serotonin syndrome," which includes agitation, anxiety, restlessness, hyperthermia, rapid heart rate, sweating, muscle tightness or rigidity, seizures, unconsciousness, and rarely death. Tricyclic antidepressants can cause severe anticholinergic side-effects, which is why they are no longer an initial choice to treat depression. Some tricyclic antidepressants are used to treat insomnia because of their sedative effects. Trazodone can also be highly sedating due to its antihistaminic effects.

The drugs in this chapter are largely presented in order of when each class was discovered historically.

Serotonin and norepinephrine are the principal neurotransmitters associated with depression. In general, five steps are associated with the transmission of nerve signals: 1) neurons produce neurotransmitters; 2) neurons store them until needed; 3) neurons release them when needed; 4) neurotransmitters cross the synapse and bind with a receptor on the post-synaptic neuron thus transmitting the signal; and 5) extra neurotransmitters in the synapse are removed and the presynaptic neuron is signaled to stop releasing the neurotransmitter.

ANTI-DEPRESSANTS

Depression, considered to result in part from a lack of serotonin and/or norepinephrine, is treated with drugs that increase serotonin and norepinephrine levels. Increasing serotonin and norepinephrine levels can be accomplished in several different ways exploiting the several steps involved in the production, storage, release, re-uptake, and metabolism of these two neurotransmitters.

MONOAMINE OXIDASE INHIBITORS

Isocarboxazid, phenelzine, tranylcypromine, and selegiline are MAOIs. MAOIs prevent the enzyme monoamine oxidase from metabolizing serotonin, norepinephrine, and dopamine (although dopamine is not thought to directly influence depression) into biologically inactive metabolites. Thus, MAOIs increase levels of serotonin and norepinephrine which for many patients effectively treats depression.

The enzyme monoamine oxidase has two subtypes: MAO-A and MAO-B. MAO-B is found primarily in the brain. MAO-A is found in the GI tract, liver, and in the CNS. Inhibition of MAO-A in the GI tract and liver can cause a severe increase in blood pressure called "hypertensive crisis," when administered with tyramine containing foods. All of the above drugs, except selegiline, inhibit both MAO-A and MAO-B, thus they can cause hypertensive crisis. Selegiline is used solely for Parkinson's disease (included here for comparison purposes). Selegiline selectively inhibits MAO-B at low doses.

Despite their effectiveness, MAOIs are rarely used today because of their side-effects and innumerable drug interactions and food interactions (red wine). They are reserved for patients with depression who do not respond to newer treatments.

Side-effects

Hypertensive crisis is the most severe adverse effect resulting from the use of MAOIs. MAOIs prevent the metabolism of other drugs and/or tyramine (found in red wine), either of which often results in hypertensive crisis, a medical emergency. Selegiline, a selective inhibitor for MAO-B, is unlikely to cause a hypertensive crisis as long as normal doses are used.

Drug Interactions

MAOIs inhibit the metabolism of SSRIs, SNRIs, TCAs, and bupropion (among many other drugs). These drugs should not be used in combination with MAOIs. MAOIs, when given with SSRIs, TCAs, and SNRIs can cause serotonin syndrome. Serotonin syndrome can cause agitation, restlessness, anxiety, diarrhea, muscle twitches, rigidity, seizures, and unconsciousness. Sometimes, serotonin syndrome can be fatal.

TRICYCLIC ANTIDEPRESSANTS

Amitriptyline, clomipramine, doxepin, imipramine, amoxapine, desipramine, maprotiline, nortriptyline, and protriptyline are tricyclic antidepressants. TCAs work by inhibiting presynaptic neurons from re-uptaking serotonin and norepinephrine back into the presynaptic neuron. The reuptake of serotonin and norepinephrine is the primary means of ending neurotransmission. By blocking the reuptake of serotonin and norepinephrine, there is more of them to stimulate postsynaptic receptors, which may decrease depression in some patients.

TCAs are not the first choice of most clinicians. Their considerable side-effects, notably anticholinergic effects including dry mouth, constipation, and potential arrhythmias, relegate them to use after a patient has tried a selective serotonin reuptake inhibitor. TCAs are used to treat neuropathic pain, headaches, and insomnia. They are much cheaper than newer insomnia medications.

Side-effects

TCAs are structurally similar to both antihistamines and anticholinergic drugs. Consequently, TCAs cause severe sedation resulting from their similarity to antihistamines. Because of their structural similarity to anticholinergic drugs, TCA's cause dry mouth, blurred vision, difficultly with urinating, and tachycardia (remember the anticholinergic drug atropine increases heart rate). TCAs also cause orthostatic hypotension, weight gain, and sedation.

Drug Interactions

The co-administration of TCAs with other drugs that have antihistamine properties or anticholinergic properties increases the side-effects of each. Some TCAs are metabolized by CYP2D6. Inhibitors of CYP2D6 can increase levels of TCAs.

SELECTIVE SEROTONIN REUPTAKE INHIBITORS

Sertraline, fluoxetine, citalopram fluvoxamine, and escitalopram are commonly used selective serotonin reuptake inhibitors (SSRIs). Presynaptic neurons release serotonin and then reuptake or recover serotonin once it has had a chance to activate post-synaptic neurons. SSRIs prevent presynaptic neurons from reuptaking serotonin, thus making more serotonin available to bind with receptors on the postsynaptic neuron; thus lessening the symptoms of depression. Specifically, SSRIs block the serotonin transporter (SERT). SERT is a protein located on presynaptic nerve endings that removes serotonin from the synapse between nerves and returns it to the presynaptic nerve.

Side-effects

As a class, SSRIs are well tolerated. SSRIs are much better tolerated than TCAs, and therefore have largely replaced TCAs as first line therapy. Serotonin syndrome occurs in very few patients. Serotonin syndrome includes agitation, anxiety, restlessness, hyperthermia, rapid heart rate, sweating, muscle tightness or rigidity, seizures, unconsciousness, and rarely death. Other side-effects include drowsiness, insomnia, anxiety (despite being used to treat anxiety), delayed ejaculation, nausea, and vomiting. SSRIs can increase the risk of suicidal thinking and behavior (suicidality) in children, adolescents, young adults (18-24).

Drug Interactions

In general, SSRIs inhibit CYP2D6. Thus, they block the metabolism of drugs depending on CYP2D6 for metabolism. Perhaps most importantly, inhibiting CYP2D6 prevents the liver from converting tamoxifen, a breast cancer drug, into its active metabolite. Fluvoxamine inhibits CYP3A4.

SSRIs are themselves partially metabolized by monoamine oxidase; consequently, MAOIs prevent MAO from metabolizing of SSRIs. SSRIs should not be used until 14 days after a MAOI has been stopped.

SEROTONIN-NOREPINEPHRINE REUPTAKE INHIBITORS

Serotonin-norepinephrine reuptake inhibitors (SNRIs) block both the serotonin transporter (SERT) and the norepinephrine transporter (NET) from transporting serotonin and norepinephrine, respectively, back into the presynaptic neurons that originally released them into the synaptic cleft. Desvenlafaxine, duloxetine, milnacipran, and venlafaxine are SNRIs available in the U.S. Duloxetine is approved to treat major depressive disorder (MDD), generalized anxiety disorder (GAD), diabetic peripheral neuropathic pain (DPNP), fibromyalgia (FM), and chronic musculoskeletal pain. Venlafaxine is approved to treat major depressive disorder, generalized anxiety disorder, social anxiety disorder, and panic disorder. Milnacipran is approved to treat fibromyalgia. Desvenlafaxine is approved to treat major depressive disorder.

Side-effects

As with SSRIs, SNRIs are capable of causing serotonin syndrome. Additionally, SSRIs and SNRIs can increase the risk of suicidal thinking and behavior (suicidality) in children, adolescents, and young adults (18-24). Similar to SSRIs, SNRIs can cause nausea and delayed ejaculation. Additionally, SNRIs can aggravate narrow-angle glaucoma.

Drug Interactions

SNRIs are contraindicated with MAOIs; patients must be free from a MAOI for 14 days before starting a SNRI. Duloxetine is a major substrate of both CYP1A2 and CYP2D6; consequently, any drug that inhibits CYP2D6 or CYP1A2 will increase blood levels of duloxetine. Drugs that induce CYP2D6 or CYP1A2 will decrease blood levels of duloxetine.

Venlafaxine is a major substrate of both CYP2D6 and CYP3A4. Inhibitors or inducers of either will alter venlafaxine blood levels. Desvenlafaxine may interfere with warfarin, potentially increasing bleeding. Desvenlafaxine is not a substrate for P-glycoprotein. Serotonin syndrome may result from the coadministration of milnacipran, venlafaxine, or desvenlafaxine with other drugs that affect serotonin. Triptans (migraine drugs), anti-psychotics, and dopamine antagonists may increase serotonin levels, despite that not being their main mechanism of action.

ATYPICAL ANTIDEPRESSANTS

Bupropion is a weak inhibitor of the reuptake of dopamine and norepinephrine back into presynaptic neurons. It is approved to treat major depressive disorder. Bupropion is contraindicated in patients with seizure disorders, bulimia, or anorexia nervosa. It is also contraindicated in patients undergoing abrupt withdrawal of alcohol or sedatives (including benzodiazepines). Finally, bupropion must not be started until 14 days after cessation of a MAOI. It is metabolized by CYP2B6. It also inhibits CYP2D6.

Mirtazapine is an antagonist at central presynaptic alpha-2 adrenergic inhibitory auto-receptors and hetero-receptors. This putatively increases central noradrenergic and serotonergic activity. Mirtazapine is also an antagonist at 5-HT-2 and 5-HT-3 receptors, although this does not play a role in its anti-depressive properties. Mirtazapine is approved to treat major depressive disorder. As with other antidepressants, patients must be off MAOIs for at least 14 days before starting mirtazapine. Mirtazapine, because it is structurally similar to antihistamines, causes severe sedation. It is metabolized by CYP2D6, CYP1A2, and CYP3A4.

Trazodone is approved to treat major depressive disorder. Trazodone selectively inhibits neuronal reuptake of serotonin and is an antagonist at 5-HT-2A/2C serotonin receptors. Trazodone causes postural hypotension; a result of its antagonism at alpha-1 adrenergic receptors. As with other antidepressants, trazodone may increase the risk of suicide in children, adolescents, and young adults (18-24). It is metabolized by CYP3A4. The kidneys eliminate 70-75% of an oral dose within 72 hours of ingestion. Because of its similarity to antihistamines, trazodone is quite sedating.

Monoamine Oxidase Inhibitors				
Generic Name / Brand Name	Clinical Use / Contraindications	Dose	Dosage Form	Mechanism of Action
Phenelzine Nardil®	Depressed patients who have been clinically characterized as "atypical." Contraindications: pheochromocytoma, congestive heart failure, severe renal impairment or renal disease, history of liver disease, abnormal liver function tests, sympathomimetic drugs, aged cheeses, salami, yogurt, excessive caffeine, chocolate, dextromethorphan, or alcohol.	Adult initial oral dose: 15 mg 3 times daily, maintenance dose: 15 mg a day or every other day	Generic tablet: 15 mg; Nardil® tablet: 15 mg	Irreversibly inhibits both MAO-A and MAO-B, thus preventing the metabolism of dopamine, norepinephrine, and serotonin
Tranylcypromine Parnate®	Major Depressive Episode Without Melancholia. Rarely should it be the first antidepressant that a patient uses. Contraindications: Cerebrovascular defects, cardiovascular disorders, pheochromocytoma, tricyclic antidepressants.	Adult oral dose: 10 mg three times daily	Generic tablet: 10 mg; Parnate® tablet: 10 mg	Irreversibly inhibits both MAO-A and MAO-B, thus preventing the metabolism of dopamine, norepinephrine, and serotonin.

Tricyclic Antidepressants				
Generic Name / Brand Name	Clinical Use/ Contraindications	Dose	Dosage Form	Mechanism of Action
Amitriptyline Elavil®	Depression Contraindications: MAO-I within 14 days; immediately after heart attack because of heart block.	Start adults at: 50-150 mg a day in divided doses or as a single bedtime dose. Usual maintenance range: 50-300 mg a day in divided doses.	Generic tablets: 10, 25, 50, 75, 100, and 150 mg	Inhibits the pre-synaptic reuptake of serotonin and norepinephrine
Amoxapine Asendin	Depression Contraindications: avoid using within 14 days of a MAOI.	Starting adult dose: 50 mg two to three times daily. Usual maintenance dose: 200-300 mg a day. Max dose of 400 mg a day.	Generic tablets: 25, 50, 100, and 150 mg	Same as above
Clomipramine Anafranil®	Depression and obsessive-compulsive disorder. Contraindications: use of clomipramine and a MAOI within 14 days of each other. Do not use with linezolid, intravenous methylene blue.	Start at 25 mg daily. If necessary, gradually increase dose to 100 mg during first 14 days. If necessary, may increase dose again over 2 more weeks to 250 mg daily.	Generic and Anafranil® capsules: 25, 50, and 75 mg	Same as above
Desipramine Norpramin®	Depression Contraindications: Avoid using within 14 days of MAOI. Do not use with linezolid, intravenous methylene blue.	Usual adult dose is 100 mg to 200 mg daily. Severely ill patients may need 300 mg daily. Doses above 300 mg are not recommended.	Generic tablets and Norpramin®: 10, 25, 50, 75, 100, and 150 mg	Inhibits the pre-synaptic reuptake of serotonin and norepinephrine
Doxepin Sinequan®, Silenor®	Psychoneurotic patients with depression and/or anxiety. Depression and/or anxiety associated with alcoholism (not to be taken while patient is still drinking). Psychotic depressive disorders associated with anxiety. Contraindications: Do not use within 14 days of a MAOI. Glaucoma, tendency to urinary retention.	Start most patients at 75 mg daily. Usual dose range is 75 mg to 150 mg daily. Some patients may need 300 mg daily.	Generic capsules: 10, 25, 50, 75, 100, and 150 mg; Oral solution: 10 mg/ml 118 and 120 ml containers; Silenor® tablets: 3 and 6 mg	Same as above and an antagonist at H-1 receptors

Tricyclic Antidepressants				
Generic Name / Brand Name	Clinical Use/ Contraindications	Dose	Dosage Form	Mechanism of Action
Imipramine Tofranil, Tofranil PM	Depression; nocturnal enuresis Contraindications: same as above	Start at 25 mg to 75 mg daily at bedtime. Usual range is 150 mg to 300 mg PO at bedtime.	Generic and Tofranil tablets: 10, 25, and 50 mg; generic capsules and Tofranil-PM: 75, 100, 125, and 150 mg	Inhibits the pre-synaptic reuptake of serotonin and norepinephrine
Maprotiline Ludiomil	Major depressive disorder; anxiety with depression Contraindications: same as above	Usual starting dose: 75 mg daily. Usual maintenance range: 75 mg to 150 mg.	Generic tablet: 25, 50, and 75 mg	Same as above
Nortriptyline Pamelor®	Depression Contraindications: do not use within 14 days of a MAOI. Do not use with linezolid, methylene blue, do not use during acute recovery time after myocardial infarction.	Usual adult dose: 25 mg three to four times daily. Usual maintenance range of 75 mg to 150 mg. Doses above 150 mg are not recommended.	Generic and Pamelor® capsules: 10, 25, 50 and 75 mg; Oral Solution: 10 mg/5ml	Same as above
Protriptyline Vivactil®	Depression Contraindications: Same as above	Usual starting adult dose: 15-60 mg a day. Maintenance dose: 15-60 mg a day.	Generic and Vivactil® tablets: 5 and 10 mg	Same as above

Selective Serotonin Reuptake Inhibitors				
Generic Name / Brand Name	Clinical Use/ Contraindications	Dose	Dosage Form	Mechanism of Action
Citalopram Celexa®	Depression Contraindications: avoid using with 14 days of a MAOI. Do not use with linezolid, or methylene blue.	Initial adult dose: 20 mg once daily. Max increase to 40 mg daily after one week. Doses above 40 mg are not recommended because of QT prolongation.	Generic tablets: 10, 20, and 40 mg; Celexa® tablets: 10, 20, and 40 mg	Selectively blocks the presynaptic reuptake of serotonin

Selective Serotonin Reuptake Inhibitors				
Generic Name / Brand Name	Clinical Use/ Contraindications	Dose	Dosage Form	Mechanism of Action
Escitalopram Lexapro®	Acute and maintenance treatment of Major Depressive Disorder. Acute treatment of Generalized Anxiety Disorder. Contraindications: Do not use within 14 days of a MAOI. Do not use with linezolid, methylene blue, or pimozide.	Initial adult or adolescents dose for MDD is 10 mg once daily. Usual maintenance dose of 10 mg once daily. Maximum of 20 mg once daily. Adult dose of GAD is 10 mg once daily. Not indicated for GAD in adolescents.	Tablet: 5, 10, and 20 mg; Lexapro® Oral Solution: 1 mg/ml 240 ml container	Selectively blocks the presynaptic reuptake of serotonin
Fluoxetine Prozac®, Prozac® Weekly, Sarafem®	Major depressive disorder; Bulimia Nervosa, obsessive-compulsive disorder, premenstrual dysphoric disorder; and panic disorder. Contraindications: Do not use MAOI within 5 weeks of stopping fluoxetine. Do not start fluoxetine within 14 days of stopping an MAOI. Do not use with linezolid, methylene blue, or pimozide.	Adult major depressive disorder, initial oral dose: 20 mg once daily in the morning. Usual maintenance range: 20 mg to 40 mg daily. Max of 80 mg daily.	Generic and Prozac® capsules: 10, 20, and 40 mg; Prozac® Weekly delayed release capsule: 90 mg; generic tablets: 10 and 20 mg; generic oral solution: 20 mg/5 ml	Same as above
Fluvoxamine Luvox® CR	Obsessive-compulsive disorder Contraindications: Do not use within 14 days of an MAOI. Avoid using with linezolid or methylene blue.	Recommend starting dose is 50 mg once daily at bedtime. May increase by 50 mg a day at 4 to7 day intervals if needed. Max dose of 300 mg daily. Doses over 100 mg daily need to be divided.	Generic tablets: 25, 50, and 100 mg; Luvox® CR capsule: 100 and 150 mg	Same as above

Selective Serotonin Reuptake Inhibitors				
Generic Name / Brand Name	Clinical Use/ Contraindications	Dose	Dosage Form	Mechanism of Action
Paroxetine Paxil®, Paxil® CR	Major depressive disorder; obsessive-compulsive disorder; panic disorder; social anxiety disorder; generalized anxiety disorder; post-traumatic stress disorder. Contraindications: Do not use within 14 days of a MAOI. Thioridazine, pimozide.	For major depressive disorder the initial adult dose is 20 mg once daily, with or without food, generally in the morning.	Generic and Paxil® tablets: 10, 20, 30, and 40 mg; Generic extended release tablets and Paxil® CR: 12.5, 25, and 37.5 mg; Oral Suspension: 10 mg/5 ml 250 ml container	Same as above
Sertraline Zoloft®	Major Depressive Disorder; Obsessive-compulsive disorder; Panic disorder; post-traumatic stress disorder; premenstrual dysphoric disorder; social anxiety disorder. Contraindications: Do not use within 14 days of a MAOI. Do not use with linezolid, methylene blue, or pimozide.	Major depressive disorder: adult dose of 50 mg once daily. Panic disorder, post-traumatic stress disorder, and social anxiety disorder adult doses should be initiated at 25 mg once daily, after a week increase to 50 mg once daily. Premenstrual dysphoric disorder initiate dose at 50 mg once daily either through out the menstrual cycle or limited to the luteal phase, based on clinician's assessment.	Generic and Zoloft® tablets: 25, 50, and 100 mg; generic and Zoloft® oral solution: 20 mg/ml 60 ml container	Same as above

Serotonin and Norepinephrine Reuptake Inhibitors				
Generic Name / Brand Name	Clinical Use/ Contraindications	Dose	Dosage Form	Mechanism of Action
Desvenlafaxine Pristiq®	Major depressive disorder. Contraindications: Do not use MAOIs within 7 days of stopping desvenlafaxine. Do not use desvenlafaxine within 14 days of stopping a MAOI.	50 mg once daily with or without food. Doses above 50 mg are probably not effective.	Pristiq® tablets: 50 and 100 mg	Inhibits the presynaptic reuptake of both serotonin and norepinephrine

Serotonin and Norepinephrine Reuptake Inhibitors				
Generic Name / Brand Name	Clinical Use/ Contraindications	Dose	Dosage Form	Mechanism of Action
Duloxetine Cymbalta®	Major depressive disorder; GAD; diabetic peripheral neuropathic pain; fibromyalgia; chronic muscloskeletal pain Contraindications: do not use MAOI within 5 days of stopping duloxetine. Do not use duloxetine within 14 days of stopping a MAOI.	Adult initial oral dose for major depressive disorder: 40-60 mg once daily. Target dose of 40 mg (20 mg twice daily) to 60 mg daily (30 mg twice daily, or 60 mg once daily).	Cymbalta® capsules: 20, 30, and 60 mg	Inhibits the presynaptic reuptake of both serotonin and norepinephrine, weakly inhibits reuptake of dopamine
Milnacipran Savella®	Fibromyalgia Contraindications: Do not use within 14 days of stopping a MAOI.	Day 1: 12.5 mg once Days 2-3: 12.5 mg BID Days 4-7: 25 mg BID After day 7: 50 mg BID Maintenance dose 50 mg BID	Savella® titration pack: 12.5 mg, 25 mg, and 50 mg tablets; Savella® tablets: 12.5, 25, 50, and 100 mg	Inhibits serotonin and norepinephrine presynaptic reuptake
Venlafaxine Effexor®, Effexor® XR	Major depressive disorder Contraindications: Do not use within 14 days of stopping a MAOI. Do not use a MAOI within 7 days of stopping venlafaxine. Do not use with linezolid or methylene blue.	Recommended starting dose is 75 mg divided in 2 or 3 doses, with food. If necessary, may increase to 150 mg daily. If needed, may then increase to 225 mg daily. Increase dose at intervals of 4 days. Max dose of 225 mg daily for outpatients. Some hospitalized patients used 350 mg daily.	Generic tablet: 25, 37.5, 50, 75, and 100 mg; generic and Effexor® XR capsules: 37.5, 75, and 150 mg; generic extended release tablets: 37.5, 75, 150, and 225 mg	Same as above

Atypical Antidepressants				
Generic Name / Brand Name	Clinical Use/ Contraindications	Dose	Dosage Form	Mechanism of Action
Buproprion Wellbutrin®	Major depressive disorder (MDD); adjunct for quitting smoking Contraindications: seizure disorders, Zyban®, bulimia, anorexia nervosa, abrupt discontinuation of alcohol. Do not use within 14 days of stopping a MAOI.	Initial adult dose: 100 mg BID. Usual adult maintenance dose of 100 mg TID if needed.	Generic and Wellbutrin® tablets: 75 and 100 mg; generic and Wellbutrin® SR: 100, 150, 200 mg; generic and Wellbutrin® XL: 150 and 300 mg	Inhibits reuptake of norepinephrine and dopamine; thought to promote the pre-synaptic release of norepinephrine and dopamine
Mirtazapine Remeron®	Major Depressive Disorder Contraindications: do not use within 14 days of a MAOI. Do not start an MAOI until 14 days after stopping mirtazapine.	Recommended starting adult dose is 15 mg QD, usually in the evening before bedtime.	Generic tablets: 7.5, 15, 30, and 45 mg; Remeron® tablets: 15, 30, and 45 mg; Remeron® SolT-ab: 15, 30, and 45 mg	Antagonist at central alpha-2 presynaptic receptors, thus blocking the negative feedback loop, thus increasing the concentration of serotonin and norepinephrine in the synaptic cleft
Trazodone Desyrel®, Oleptro®	Major depressive disorder Contraindications: Do not use within 14 days of a MAOI. Do not use MAOI within 7 days of stopping trazodone.	Usual staring adult dose is 50 mg TID. Usual range maintenance range is 150 mg to 300 mg daily in divided doses.	Generic tablets: 50, 100, 150, and 300 mg; Oleptro® extended release tablets: 150 and 300 mg	Inhibits the presynaptic reuptake of serotonin; blocks alpha-1 receptors

CHAPTER 6

ANTIPSYCHOTICS

Typical Antipsychotics (1st generation)	Atypical Antipsychotics (2nd generation)
Chlorpromazine Perphenazine Trifluoperazine Fluphenazine Thiothixene Thioridazine Prochlorperazine Loxapine Haloperidol	Aripiprazole Clozapine Iloperidone Olanzapine Paliperidone Quetiapine Risperidone Ziprasidone

Excess dopamine is believed to cause schizophrenia. Typical and atypical antipsychotics are antagonists at the dopamine D_2 receptor. Atypical antipsychotics are also antagonists at the $5\text{-}HT_2$ receptor. Atypical antipsychotics cause less parkinsonism, akathisia, tardive dyskinesia, and dystonia than the typical antipsychotics cause. Aripiprazole, seroquel and iloperidone may cause orthostatic hypotension by antagonism at alpha$_1$ receptors. Antipsychotics can prolong the QT interval. Because the atypicals cause less side-effects, patients may be more compliant with them. Olanzapine is rarely used anymore because of its side-effects including hyperglycemia, hyperlipidemia, and weight gain.

Both classes are typically dosed once to twice daily. Many atypical antipsychotics are available as injections and sublingual tablets because some older patients and younger patients are unable to swallow tablets.

Psychosis is a disconnection with reality. Treatment depends on the cause. Psychosis can result from a variety of causes including illicit drugs, schizophrenia, mania, dementia, delirium, Alzheimer's, and side-effects of drugs used to treat other diseases (levodopa used to treat Parkinson's). In Alzheimer's, psychosis results from loss of neurons that release acetylcholine. Treatment with acetylcholinesterase inhibitors may be beneficial in Alzheimer's. Anticholinergic drugs may worsen psychosis caused by Alzheimer's. In Parkinson's, levodopa therapy may cause psychosis. Psychosis stemming from delirium can result from anticholinergic drugs, electrolyte imbalances, infection, and metabolic problems.

Psychosis caused by dementia can be worsened by anticholinergic drugs. Consequently, antipsychotics with the least anticholinergic properties are preferred to treat this form of psychosis. Haloperidol, a first generation antipsychotic, and risperidone, a second generation antipsychotic, have the least anticholinergic properties. Although, it should be kept in mind that neither risperidone, nor haloperidol are officially approved to treat psychosis caused by dementia, clinicians do often use them for this purpose despite a black box warning that they increase the risk of death. Because of the risk of side-effects, doses for the elderly are usually much lower than doses for younger patients.

Schizophrenia and its related disorders are thought to result from an excess of dopamine binding with D_2 receptors in the mesolimbic area of the brain. Other receptors probably influence schizophrenia as well. Schizophrenia causes positive symptoms and negative symptoms. Positive symptoms include lack-of-movement disorders, thought disorders, delusions, and hallucinations. Negative symptoms include lack of enjoyment of life, flat affect (absence of facial features, dull or monotonous voice), and diminished speaking. Another common symptom of psychotic disorders is decreased cognitive functioning including, decreased ability to focus and poor decision making.

Two different classes of antipsychotic drugs have been developed to treat schizophrenia. Both classes block dopamine at D_2 receptors thus lessening psychosis. The typical antipsychotics (also called first generation) cause severe side-effects. Atypical antipsychotics (also called second generation) usually cause less side-effects than typical antipsychotics.

TYPICAL ANTIPSYCHOTICS

The typical antipsychotics all have similar therapeutic effectiveness at treating schizophrenia. Chlorpromazine is approved to treat mania and schizophrenia, among other non-psychosis related indications. Also, it is commonly used to treat psychosis and agitation that are secondary to Alzheimer's dementia. Chlorpromazine, as do other antipsychotics, carries a black box warning for increased risk of death for elderly patients with dementia-related psychosis, when compared with placebo. Perphenazine, trifluoperazine, fluphenazine, thiothixene, thioridazine, prochlorperazine, loxapine, and haloperidol are typical antipsychotics.

Side-effects

Because of its chemical structure, chlorpromazine mimics antihistamines, anticholinergics, and alpha blockers; consequently, it causes sedation, anticholinergic effects (drowsiness, dry mouth, constipation etc), and orthostasis. Chlorpromazine is also known to cause life-threatening arrhythmias, QT prolongation, and torsades de pointes. All antipsychotic medications can prolong the QT interval of the heart; sometimes torsades de pointes and ventricular arrhythmias may result from antipsychotic use.

Although rare, neuroleptic malignant syndrome (NMS) may result from use of typical antipsychotics, especially haloperidol. NMS symptoms include fever, muscular rigidity, and mental stupor, and autonomic dysfunction, among many other symptoms. Haloperidol also causes considerable sedation. Weight gain is a common side-effect of antipsychotic medications.

Drug Interactions

They should not be combined with other drugs that also cause QT prolongation or torsades de pointes. Further, because of the severe sedation, anticholinergic effects, and lowered blood pressure, be careful using these drugs with other drugs that are also sedating, anticholinergic, and lower blood pressure.

ATYPICAL ANTIPSYCHOTICS

The atypical antipsychotics, aripiprazole, clozapine, olanzapine, quetiapine, risperidone, and ziprasidone, treat schizophrenia and other forms of psychosis. All are antagonists at the D_2 receptor and $5\text{-}HT_2$ receptor.

Both the typical and atypical antipsychotics are considered to have equal efficacy. Regarding the "negative symptoms" of schizophrenia, patients respond better to risperidone than the typical antipsychotics. The atypicals generally cause fewer side-effects than the typicals.

As, antagonists at the $5\text{-}HT_2$ receptor, they benefit patients who are non-responsive to standard SSRI therapy; exactly why is unknown. When newer atypical antipsychotics ($5\text{-}HT_2$ antagonists) are combined with an SSRI, patients who previously did not respond to the SSRI, now respond to it. In fact, olanzapine is available with fluoxetine in a single dosage unit. Olanzapine is rarely used anymore because of its side-effects including hyperglycemia, hyperlipidemia, and weight gain. However, aripiprazole is approved as adjunctive therapy with an SSRI to treat major depressive disorder. Aripiprazole is also approved to treat bipolar I disorder.

Side-effects

The lower side-effects of the atypical antipsychotics improve patient compliance. They are less potent antagonists at dopamine D-2 receptors than the typical antipsychotics. This causes less extrapyramidal side-effects, parkinsonism, akathisia, tardive dyskinesia, and dystonia. Clozapine causes seizures and agranulocytosis in about 1% of patients (patients must have frequent lab tests). Further, clozapine and olanzapine can cause diabetes. Because of these side-effects, these two are rarely used. The atypicals have little anticholinergic side-effects because their structures differ from cholinergic antagonists.

The atypical antipsychotics all have black box warnings concerning sudden death in elderly patients. Elderly patients with dementia-related psychosis have a higher risk of death when using atypical antipsychotics relative to placebo. This includes heart failure, sudden death or infection (pneumonia). In addition, aripiprazole and seroquel may cause orthostatic hypotension by antagonism at $alpha_1$ receptors.

Drug Interactions

Inducers of CYP3A4 such as phenytoin, carbamazepine, rifampin, and barbiturates decrease blood levels of aripiprazole. In contrast, the CYP3A4 inhibitor, ketoconazole, substantially increases aripiprazole's and iloperidone's blood levels. Further, fluoxetine, an inhibitor of CYP2D6, increases blood levels of aripiprazole and clozapine.

Typical Antipsychotics

Dosing principles: always use the smallest effective dose; adjust doses based on severity of symptoms; generally avoid exceeding the manufacturer's recommended maximum dose because higher doses do not usually produce beneficial results.

Generic Name / Brand Name	Clinical Use/ Contraindications	Dose	Dosage Form	Mechanism of Action
Chlorpromazine Thorazine®	Manages psychotic disorders such as mania and schizophrenia; nausea and vomiting Contraindications: CNS depressants, CNS depression, Parkinsons' disease	Starting adult dose of 10 mg -25 mg TID. May increase if needed.	Generic tablets: 10, 25, 50, 100, and 200 mg; solution for injection: 25 mg/ml 1 and 2 ml vials	Antagonist at the D_2 receptor, thus preventing dopamine from binding
Fluphenazine Prolixin®	Psychotic disorders; schizophrenia Contraindications: severe CNS depression, coma, blood dyscrasias, liver damage	Adult initial dose 0.5 mg to 10 mg daily in divided doses, 3 to 4 times daily.	Generic tablets: 1, 2.5, 5, and 10 mg; Oral elixir: 2.5 mg/5ml; Decanoate oil for injection: 25 mg/ml; solution for injection: 2.5 mg/ml	Antagonist at D_1 and D_2 receptors
Haloperidol Haldol®	Schizophrenia; Tourette's disorder Contraindications: same as above	Starting adult PO dose for schizophrenia: 0.5-5mg 2 to 3 times daily.	Generic tablets: 0.5, 1, 2, 5, 10, and 20 mg; oral solution: 2 mg/ml; solution for injection: 5 mg/ml.	Antagonist at D_1 and D_2 receptors
Loxapine Loxitane®	Psychotic disorders Contraindications: same as above	Starting adult PO dose: 10 mg BID.	Generic and Loxitane® capsules: 5, 10, 25, and 50 mg	Antagonist at $5\text{-}HT_{1A}$ receptor
Perphenazine Trilafon®	Schizophrenia; severe nausea and vomiting Contraindications: comatose or severely obese patients; large doses of CNS depressants; blood dyscrasias, bone marrow depression, or liver damage.	Individualize doses based on the patient. Non-hospitalized patients 4 mg to 8 mg TID initially, then reduce as soon as possible to lowest effective dosage.	Generic tablets: 2, 4, 8, and 16 mg	Antagonist at the D_2 receptor, thus preventing dopamine from binding

Typical Antipsychotics				
Dosing principles: always use the smallest effective dose; adjust doses based on severity of symptoms; generally avoid exceeding the manufacturer's recommended maximum dose because higher doses do not usually produce beneficial results.				
Generic Name / Brand Name	Clinical Use/ Contraindications	Dose	Dosage Form	Mechanism of Action
Prochlorperazine Compazine®	Schizophrenia; generalized anxiety; severe nausea and vomiting Contraindications: known sensitivity to phenothiazines; comatose; CNS depressants, alcohol, barbiturates	Outpatients psychotic disorders: 5 mg to 10 mg 3 to 4 times daily for mild conditions. For moderate to severe conditions use 10 mg 3 to 4 times daily.	Generic tablets: 5 and 10 mg; Rectal suppository generic and Compro: 25 mg; Solution for injection: 5 mg/ml 2 and 10 ml	Antagonist at D_1 and D_2 postsynaptic receptors
Trifluoperazine Stelazine®	Schizophrenia Contraindications: CNS depressions, CNS depressants	Starting adult PO dose for non-hospitalized patients: 1-2 mg twice daily; hospitalized patients: upto 40 mg a day	Generic tablets: 1, 2, 5, and 10 mg	Antagonist at the D_2 receptor, thus preventing dopamine from binding
Thiothixene Navane®	Schizophrenia Contraindications: circulatory collapse, comatose states, CNS depression, or blood dyscrasias.	Patients 12 years of age and older: recommended initial dose 2 mg three times daily. If needed, may increase to 15 mg daily in divided doses.	Generic capsules: 1, 2, 5, and 10 mg	Antagonist at D_2 receptors
Thioridazine Mellaril	Schizophrenia Contraindications: severe hypertension, cardiovascular disease, liver damage	Starting adult PO dose: 50-100 mg three times daily. Maintenance dose: may slowly increase dose if needed, max dose of 800 mg a day in divided doses	Generic tablets: 10, 25, 50, and 100 mg	Antagonist at postsynaptic D_2 receptors in mesolimbic area

Atypical Antipsychotics				
Generic Name / Brand Name	Clinical Use/ Contraindications:	Dose	Dosage Form	Mechanism of Action
Aripiprazole Abilify®	Schizophrenia; bipolar I disorder; adjunctive treatment for major depressive disorder. Contraindications: known sensitivity to aripiprazole.	Initial adult PO dose for schizophrenia: 10-15 mg once daily. Max dose of 30 mg daily for all indications.	Abilify® tablets: 2, 5, 10, 15, 20, 30 mg	A partial agonist at both D_2 and $5\text{-}HT_{1A}$ receptors; antagonist at $5\text{-}HT_{2A}$ receptors

Atypical Antipsychotics				
Generic Name / Brand Name	Clinical Use/ Contraindications:	Dose	Dosage Form	Mechanism of Action
Clozapine Clozaril® FazaClo®	Treatment-resistant schizophrenia Contraindications: myeloproliferative disorders, uncontrolled epilepsy, paralytic ileus, severe granulocytopenia.	Starting adult PO dose: 12.5 mg one to two times daily. Maintenance dose: may increase dose by 25-50 mg/day, if well tolerated, over 2 weeks to a range of 300-450 mg/day	Generic tablets: 25, 50, 100, and 200 mg; Clozaril® tablets: 25 and 100 mg	Antagonist at D_1, D_2, D_3, and D_5 receptors; antagonist at $5\text{-}HT_2$ alpha receptors, and H_1, and cholinergic receptors
Iloperidone Fanapt®	Schizophrenia Contraindications: known hypersensitivity to iloperidone or the inactive ingredients.	Adult initial oral dose: 1 mg BID on day 1, then 2 mg, 4 mg, 6 mg, 8 mg, 10 mg, and 12 mg BID on days 2, 3, 4, 5, 6, and 7 respectively to reach the 12 mg/day to 24 mg/day range.	Fanapt® tablets: 1, 2, 4, 6, 8, 10, and 12 mg	Antagonists at D_2 and $5\text{-}HT_2$ receptors
Olanzapine Zyprexa®	Schizophrenia Contraindications: known hypersensitivity to olanzapine or the inactive ingredients.	Initial adult PO dose: 5-10 mg once daily. Maintenance dose: 10 mg QD. Increase dose at 7 days intervals by 5 mg.	Generic and Zyprexa® tablets: 2.5, 5, 7.5, 10, 15, and 20 mg	Antagonist at D_2, $5\text{-}HT_{2A}$, $5\text{-}HT_{2C}$, H_1, and alpha$_1$ receptors
Paliperidone Invega® Invega Sustenna®	Schizophrenia; schizo-affective disorder Contraindications: known hypersensitivity to paliperidone or the inactive ingredients.	Initial adult PO dose for schizophrenia: 6 mg daily. Recommended dose: 3-12 mg a day. Max dose of 12 mg daily.	Invega® tablets: 1.5, 3, 6, and 9 mg; Invega Sustenna® suspension for injection various strengths	Antagonist at D_2 and $5\text{-}HT_{2A}$ receptors
Quetiapine Seroquel®, Seroquel XR®	Schizophrenia; acute manic episodes associated with bipolar I disorder Contraindications: known hypersensitivity to quetiapine or the inactive ingredients.	Initial adult PO dose for schizophrenia: 25 mg BID. Recommended dose range: 150-750 mg/day. Increase in increments of 25 mg to 50 mg divided 2 or 3 times on Days 2 and 3 to a range of 300 mg to 400 mg by Day 4.	Seroquel® tablets: 25, 50, 100, 200, 300, and 400 mg. Seroquel® XR: 50, 150, 200, 300, and 400 mg	Antagonist at D_2 and $5\text{-}HT_2$ receptors

Atypical Antipsychotics				
Generic Name / Brand Name	Clinical Use/ Contraindications:	Dose	Dosage Form	Mechanism of Action
Risperidone Risperdal®, Risperdal Consta®, Risperdal M-Tab®	Schizophrenia; bipolar I disorder Contraindications: known hypersensitivity to risperidone or the inactive ingredients.	Adult initial oral dose for schizophrenia: 1 mg twice daily or 2 mg once daily. Target dose: 4 to 8 mg daily. Effective dose range 4 to 16 mg.	Generic and brand tablets: 0.25, 0.5, 1, 2, 3, and 4 mg; Risperdal Consta® injection: 12.5, 25, 37.5, and 50 mg; Risperdal M-Tab® orally disintegrating: 0.5, 1, 2, 3, and 4 mg	Antagonist at D_2 and $5\text{-}HT_{2A}$ receptors
Ziprasidone Geodon®	Schizophrenia; acute treatment of bipolar I disorder Contraindications: known history of QT prolongation; recent acute myocardial infarction, uncompensated heart failure, other drugs that prolong QT interval.	Initiate schizophrenia adult po dose at 20 mg BID. Max dose of 80 mg BID. Wait at least 2 days between dose increases. Use lowest effective dose. Take with food.	Geodon® capsules: 20, 40, 60, and 80 mg; Powder for reconstitution, injection: 20 mg vial	Antagonist at D_2, $5\text{-}HT_{2A}$, and $5\text{-}HT_{1D}$ receptors; agonist at $5\text{-}HT_{1A}$ receptor

CHAPTER 7

ANTI-PARKINSON'S DRUGS

Dopamine Precursors	Dopamine Receptor Agonists	Catechol-O-Methyl Transferase (COMT) Inhibitors	Monoamine Oxidase Inhibitors (MAO-I)	Anticholinergics
Levodopa	Bromocriptine Pramipexole Ropinirole	Entacapone Tolcapone Carbidopa	Rasagiline Selegiline	Amantadine Benztropine Trihexyphenidyl

Parkinson's disease results when the dopaminergic neurons of the substantia nigra pars compacta deteriorate. The substantia nigra pars compact connects to the striatum by neurons that release dopamine in the striatum. Dopamine activates D_2 receptors. Activation of D_2 receptors in the striatum inhibits tremors. When the neurons connecting the substantia nigra to the striatum die, dopamine cannot reach the striatum where it inhibits fine motor movements; the net result is tremor of the arms and legs when they are at rest. Other problems result as well, for example, patients experience balance problems, rigidity, and an inability to move quickly (bradykinesia). Patients are treated with drugs that are turned into dopamine; drugs that activate dopamine receptors; drugs that prevent dopamine from being metabolized; and anticholinergics.

DOPAMINE PRECURSORS

Dopamine itself does not readily cross the blood-brain barrier. Therefore, patients are given levodopa, a precursor to dopamine. The enzyme aromatic amino-acid decarboxylase (AADC) converts levodopa to dopamine in both the periphery and central nervous system. AADC is so efficient at converting levodopa to dopamine that very little levodopa actually makes it across the blood-brain barrier. Consequently, an inhibitor of peripheral AADC, carbidopa, was developed. Carbidopa itself does not cross the blood-brain barrier; therefore the levodopa that crosses the blood-brain barrier can still be converted to dopamine in the central nervous system.

Overtime, patients develop resistance to levodopa therapy, resulting in necessary dose escala-

tions. Patients experience "on" periods when the drug is working and "off" periods when the drug is not working. Dyskinesias are another side-effect of levodopa therapy. They are non-controllable movements of the head, trunk, arms, and legs. They can be managed by lowering the dose of levodopa.

DOPAMINE RECEPTOR AGONISTS

As an alternative to levodopa, patients may receive dopamine receptor agonists. These include the ergot derivative bromocriptine and the non-ergot derivatives pramipexole and ropinirole. Bromocriptine activates just D_2 receptors. Ropinirole and pramipexole bind with the D_2, D_3, and D_4 receptors. Pramipexole and ropinirole can nausea, edema, and low blood pressure (dopamine dilates blood vessels), which can lead to falls. Dopamine agonists cause central nervous system side-effects including drowsiness, dreams, and hallucinations. A substantial amount of patients (40%) experience drowsiness with ropinirole; patients must be advised of this because of the possibility of causing car accidents as a result. Ropinirole also commonly causes syncope and hypotension.

COMT-INHIBITORS

Tolcapone and entacapone inhibit the enzyme catechol-o-methyl-transferase (COMT), which is responsible for metabolizing levodopa and dopamine into inactive metabolites. Entacapone, although it does not cross the blood-brain barrier, is preferred over tolcapone, because tolcapone has been associated with several reports of fatal liver toxicity. Both reduce the number of "off" periods experienced by patients.

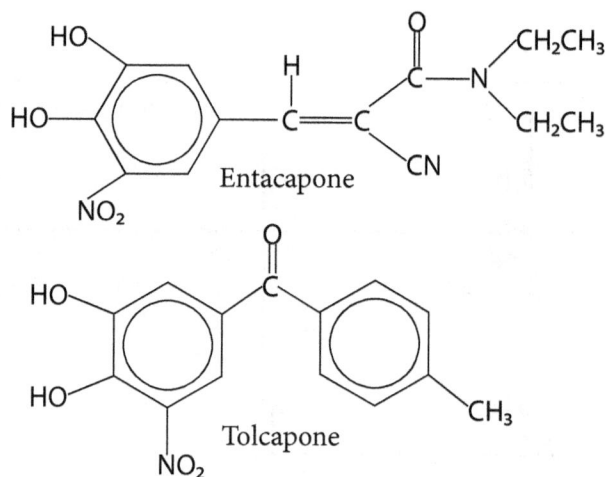

Entacapone

Tolcapone

MAO-INHIBITORS

The enzymes monoamine oxidase A (MAO-A) and monoamine oxidase B (MAO-B) both metabolize dopamine into an inactive metabolite. MAO-B is found primarily in the brain and MAO-A is found in the brain and peripheral areas of the body. Inhibitors of MAO-B and MAO-A can increase levels of dopamine in the brain, effectively treating Parkinson's disease. However, in the peripheral areas, MAO-A is responsible for metabolizing tyramine before it can cause hypertensive crisis. Thus inhibitors of MAO-A can cause hypertensive crisis if the patient consumes foods or drinks that have tyramine (red wines, legumes, etc). Selegiline is a selective inhibitor of MAO-B at normal doses. Rasagiline also selectively inhibits MAO-B. The body converts selegiline to amphetamine and methamphet-amine. Amphetamines, of course, cause sleeplessness, anxiety, and loss of appetite. Rasagiline is not converted into amphetamine or methamphetamine and hence does not have the same side-effects as selegiline.

ANTICHOLINERGICS

In addition to its slight anticholinergic properties, amantadine may stimulate dopamine release, and may block the excitatory NMDA receptors. Amantadine's therapeutic value, relative to other anti-Parkinson's drugs, is slight. It is typically used early in the disease to control movement disorders.

Trihexyphenidyl and benztropine reduce tremor through their anticholinergic properties. Acetylcholine stimulates nerves to produce muscle movement, which, when at rest, is usually counteracted by dopamine. With the loss of dopamine, acetylcholine is free to excite nerves. Blocking acetylcholine with anticholinergic drugs realigns the balance between dopamine and acetylcholine.

These three drugs share the same side-effects that other drugs with anticholinergic properties have: dry mouth, blurry vision, urinary retention, memory impairment and cognition problems. Most patients are able to withstand these side-effects, and most of them are temporary.

Therapeutic Agents for Parkinson's Disease

Generic Name / Brand Name	Use	Dose	Dosage Form	Mechanism of Action
Carbidopa Lodosyn®	Monotherapy for PD	Initial dose: 25 mg 3 to 4 times daily, maintenance doses vary based on type of levodopa product	Lodosyn® tablets 25 mg	Increases levodopa availability in the CNS by decreasing the metabolism of levodopa in the peripheral blood stream
Carbidopa and Levodopa / Sinemet® Sinemet® CR	Monotherapy for PD	Initial oral dose of immediate release tablets: carbidopa/levodopa 25/100 mg tablets, 1 tablet 3 times daily, maintenance doses: vary considerably, max dose: 200 mg of carbidopa and 2000 mg of levodopa	Generic and Sinemet® tablets: 10/100, 25/100, 25/250 carbidopa is always first and levodopa is always second	Carbidopa same as above; levodopa is converted to dopamine in the CNS
Catechol O-Methyl Transferase Inhibitors				
Entacapone Comtan®	An adjunct to carbidopa/levodopa to treat PD	One 200 mg tablet take with each levodopa/carbidopa dose. Max of 8 tablets a day.	Comtan® tablets: 200 mg	Selective and reversible inhibitor of COMT
Tolcapone Tasmar®	Adjunct to carbidopa/levodopa. If not substantially better in 3 weeks, then D/C drug	Initial dose: 100 mg 3 times daily. Recommended maintenance dose: 100 mg TID	Tasmar® tablets: 100 mg	Same as above
Carbidopa, levodopa, and entacapone Stalevo®	Monotherapy for PD	Adult initial dose: 1 "stalevo® 50" tablet 3 times daily. Maintenance doses depend on patient's response to drug. Maximum of 8 tablets daily. Only administer one tablet at a time.	Stalevo® 50: levodopa 50 mg, carbidopa 12.5 mg, and entacapone 200 mg; Stalevo® 75, Stalevo® 100, Stalevo® 125, Stalevo® 150, and Stalevo® 200.	Same as above
Dopamine Agonists				
Bromocriptine / Parlodel® Parlodel® SnapTabs	Adjunct treatment to levodopa/carbidopa.	Initial dose of 1/2 to 1 2.5 mg tablet daily, take with food. May add one 2.5 mg tablet every 2 to 7 days as needed. Usual dose range of 2.5 mg to 15 mg daily.	Generic and Parlodel® capsule: 5 mg; generic tablet: 2.5 mg; Parlodel® SnapTabs (scored) 2.5 mg	Direct agonist at D_2 receptors

Therapeutic Agents for Parkinson's Disease				
Generic Name / Brand Name	Use	Dose	Dosage Form	Mechanism of Action
Pramipexole Mirapex® Mirapex® ER	Idiopathic PD; restless leg syndrome (RLS)	Initial oral dose: 0.125 mg three times daily. Maintenance dose: 1.5 mg TID. Titrate initial dose by 0.25 mg daily every 7 days.	Generic and Mirapex® tablets: 0.125, 0.25, 0.5, 0.75, 1, and 1.5 mg; Mirapex® ER tablets: 0.375, 0.75, 1.5, 2.25, 3, 3.75, and 4.5 mg	Direct agonist at D_2 receptors in the striatum
Ropinirole Requip® Requip Xl®	Idiopathic PD	Recommended starting dose is 0.25 mg three times daily. If necessary, increase dose by 0.75 mg daily in divided doses every 7 days. Doses above 24 mg daily have not been studied.	Generic tablet and Requip®: 0.25, 0.5, 1, 2, 3, 4, and 5 mg; Requip® XL tablets: 2, 4, 6, 8, and 12 mg	Same as above
Monoamine Oxidase Inhibitors				
Rasagiline Azilect®	Monotherapy for PD; adjunct therapy to levodopa	1 mg once daily as monotherapy	Azilect® tablets: 0.5 and 1 mg	Selective and irreversible inhibitor of monoamine oxidase B
Selegiline Eldepryl®	Adjunct to levodopa/ carbidopa for PD	Adult dose: 5 mg twice daily at breakfast and lunch	Generic and Eldepryl® capsule: 5 mg; generic tablet 5 mg	At low doses (10 mg daily), inhibits MAO-B, at high doses inhibits both MAO-A and MAO-B

Anticholinergics				
Generic Name / Brand Name	Use	Dose	Dosage Form	Mechanism of Action
Amantadine Symmetrel®	Adjunct treatment for PD, drug induced extrapyramidal reactions	Adult initial oral dose: 100 mg twice daily, maintenance dose: 200 mg daily	Tablet and capsule: 100 mg; oral solution: 50 mg/5ml 473 ml bottle	Promotes release of dopamine from presynaptic neurons; blocks reuptake of dopamine into presynaptic neurons
Benztropine Cogentin®	Adjunct treatment for PD, drug induced extrapyramidal reactions	Initial dose 0.5 mg to 1mg at bedtime. Usual maintenance dose is 1-2 mg daily divided in 2 to 4 doses Max of 6 mg daily.	Tablets 0.5 mg, 1 mg, 2 mg; Injection 1mg / 1ml	Block muscarinic receptors thereby decreasing acetylcholine's excitatory actions

Trihexyphenidyl / Artane	Adjunct to carbidopa/levodopa	Initial oral dose: 1 mg daily. Maintenance dose: 2-15 mg daily. Max dose of 15 mg daily.	Generic tablets: 2 and 5 mg; oral elixir: 2 mg/5ml 473 ml bottle	Antagonist muscarinic receptors, realigns the balance between cholinergic stimulation and dopaminergic inhibition, thus less shaking

Page 60

CHAPTER 8

EPILEPSY

Focal Seizures (Formerly called "partial seizures")			Primary Generalized Seizures	
1. Seizures without altered mental status 2. Seizures with altered mental status 3. Focal seizure with secondary generalization			1. Absence seizures (typical and atypical) (petit mal) 2. Myoclonic seizures 3. Tonic-clonic seizure (grand mal)	
Prolong Sodium Channel Inactivation	Inhibitors of T-type Calcium Channels (Located in nerve cell body)	Inhibitors High-Voltage-Activated (HVA) Calcium Channels (located at presynaptic nerve ending)	GABA Reuptake Inhibitors and GABA-T Inhibitors	Synaptic Vesicle Protein (SV2A)
Phenytoin Carbamazepine Lamotrigine Oxcarbazepine Topiramate Valproic Acid Lacosamide Zonisamide Rufinamide	Ethosuximide Zonisamide Valproic Acid Clonazepam	Gabapentin Pregabalin	Tiagabine Vigabatrin	Levetiracetam

Epilepsy is the medical condition of having recurrent seizures caused by a chronic neurological condition. Seizures are sudden outbursts of repetitive and hypersynchronous nerve signals (action potentials). Some known causes of epileptic seizures include genetics, brain injury, stroke, brain surgery, sclerosis, metabolic disorders, and fevers (febrile). Not all seizures are epileptic seizures; for example, seizures from illicit drug use or alcohol withdrawal are not epileptic seizures.

Seizures have been classified according to several different naming systems over the years. Presently, seizures are divided into two main classes, each of which has three subdivisions. The two main divisions are Focal Seizures and Primary Generalized Seizures. Focal seizures are divided into seizures without altered mental status; seizures with altered mental status; and focal seizure with secondary generalization. Primary generalized seizures are divided into absence seizures (petit mal); myoclonic seizure; and tonic-clonic seizure (grand mal).

PHYSIOLOGY

Normally, two main characteristics exist to prevent the unwanted spread of an action potential to other neurons; thus preventing a seizure from occurring. The first main characteristic is repolarization of the neuron after depolarization (a two step process). Repolarization is necessary because once a neuron is depolarized, it would inherently, repetitively propagate action potentials (thus causing a seizure) if a mechanism did not exist to repolarize the neuron. Repolarization occurs in a two-step manner. Initially, almost immediately after Na^+ channels open, a portion of the Na^+ channel (inactivation gate) moves over and blocks the channel - thus preventing anymore Na^+ ions from entering the cell - thus preventing further depolarization. While this is happening, K^+ channels open and allow K^+ ions to escape the cell, which causes the cell to start to repolarize; however, the K^+ ion channels remain open long enough for the cell to become hyperpolarized (the neuron cannot initiate a new action potential while hyperpolarized.) Eventually, the K^+ channels close and the cell returns to its normal polarized state. This built-in delay of about a millisecond prevents seizures from spontaneously occurring.

Second, the nervous system uses **surround inhibition** to limit hypersynchronous action potentials. Surround inhibition is when a neuron that is sending an excitatory signal to its post-synaptic neuron also sends inhibitory signals to neurons paralleling it. These inhibitory signals, usually GABA mediated, are sent, via interneurons, to prevent surrounding neurons from developing hypersynchronous action potentials.

The problem with hypersynchronous action potentials is two-fold. One, they make it difficult, if not impossible, for the brain to determine the original source of sensory stimuli. Two, synchronous action potentials may lead to a seizure. The propagation of an action potential in one particular neuron has the inherent ability to activate synchronous action potentials in surrounding neurons. Synchronous action potentials would naturally result if the nervous system did not inhibit itself with surround inhibition. Surround inhibition prevents the initiation of synchronous action potentials in nearby neurons.

PATHOPHYSIOLOGY

FOCAL SEIZURES

Focal seizures may result when surround inhibition is not working properly. Surround inhibition may be overcome by neurons that are depolarizing repetitively. Repetitive depolarization releases excessive K^+ ions into the extracellular space between neurons. These extra K^+ ions can counteract and overcome the GABA mediated surround inhibition. Excess extracellular K^+ ions leads to a buildup of intracellular K^+ ions, which makes it easier for the neuron to reach its excitatory threshold needed to conduct an action potential. A higher frequency of action potentials may lead to seizures.

Surround inhibition can also be overcome by deficiencies in the GABA mediated interneurons that connect parallel neurons. Further, surround inhibition can be compromised by persistent and excessive accumulation of Ca^{2+} ions, which, as a consequence, releases excessive excitatory neurotransmitters into the synaptic cleft. Excess excitatory neurotransmitters can overcome surround inhibition.

FOCAL SEIZURE WITH SECONDARY GENERALIZATION

Focal seizures can start in the cortical areas of the brain. These seizures can spread to the thalamus via thalamocortical projections, and, then continue to be spread to other areas of the brain, including the opposite hemisphere from where the seizure started. Focal seizures can also spread along corpus callosum to the opposite hemisphere. Focal seizures can also spread along U-fibers to adjacent areas of the cortex where the seizure started.

PRIMARY GENERALIZED SEIZURES

The causes of primary generalized seizures are not completely understood. Absence seizures involve a disruption in the normal flow of neuronal signals between the thalamus and cortex while a patient is awake. During waking hours, the thalamus sends signals to the cortex by "tonic-firing." While a person is sleeping, the thalamus changes to "burst-firing." Burst-firing allows a person to sleep undisturbed. Burst-firing is made possible by the activation of T-type Ca^{2+} channels (located on thalamic relay neurons) while a person is asleep.

As a necessary condition of absence seizures, T-type Ca^{2+} channels engage in burst-firing while a person is awake (normally they are inactivated while a person is awake). T-type Ca^{2+} channels become activated when the thalamic relay neuron becomes hyperpolarized. The reticular thalamic nucleus may hyperpolarize the thalamic relay neuron.

Presently, two types of drugs treat absence seizures. T-type Ca^{2+} channel blockers such as ethosuximide and valproic acid block the T-type Ca^{2+} channel from initiating burst-firing. Second, clonazepam, a benzodiazepine, stops the reticular thalamic nucleus (RTN) from releasing GABA onto the thalamic relay neuron (by binding at the cell body of the RTN it inactivates the RTN, stopping the release of GABA from the end of the RTN onto the thalamic relay neuron. GABA may initiate hyperpolarization which initiates burst-firing. Further, lamotrigine treats absence seizures, exactly how, remains unknown.

ANTI-EPILEPTIC DRUGS

The various causes of seizures and epilepsy ultimately allow Na^+, K^+, and Ca^{2+} channels to propagate excessive action potentials. Most anti-epileptic drugs (AEDs) work by altering, either directly or indirectly, the flow of ions (either Na^+ or Ca^{2+} Cl^-) through ion channels. Altering the flow of ions limits the ability of neurons to rapidly and continuously transmit abnormal nerve signals. Other AEDs work by mechanisms of action that are not fully understood (levetiracetam). Most AEDs have at least two different mechanisms of action, and some have three to four mechanisms of action. Continuing research will undoubtedly continue to reveal yet undiscovered mechanisms of action for some drugs. Additionally, the N-methyl-D-aspartate receptor (NMDA-R) also plays a role in epilepsy; its activation by glutamate leads to an increase in intracellular calcium ions, which may lead to seizure generation.

AEDs are primarily classified according to which ion-channel or receptor they primarily affect; and some drugs are classified based on how they affect GABA. As with all drug classes, anticonvulsant drugs can also be classified according to their chemical structures; however, this neglects the value of knowing the mechanism of action. Anticonvulsant medications can be divided into five over-arching classes:

1. Prolonging of Na^+ channel inactivation
2. Inhibitors Ca^{2+} channels: A) T-type calcium channel and B) High voltage activated calcium channel
3. GABA agonists
4. Inhibitors of glutamate receptors
5. Synaptic vesicle protein modulator (levetiracetam)

Drugs that prolong sodium channel inactivation include lamotrigine, carbamazepine, oxcarbazepine, topiramate, and phenytoin sodium. As noted above, many drugs act by several mechanisms of action. It is not always possible to tell which mechanism of action accounts for the majority of a drug's benefit. Sodium channel blockers prolong the inactivated state of sodium channels, thus decreasing the rate at which neurons can fire. Phenytoin has been used for a long time to treat focal and secondary generalized seizures.

Dosing phenytoin is problematic in many patients because it induces its own metabolism; it also induces the metabolism of other drugs. Phenytoin also has numerous side-effects. Phenytoin's side-effects include ataxia, nystagmus, gingival hyperplasia, megaloblastic anemia, and rash. It is highly bound to plasma proteins, about 95%. Because of these drawbacks, newer agents have replaced phenytoin, including lamotrigine and carbamazepine.

Carbamazepine is approved to treat partial seizures, generalized tonic-clonic seizures, and mixed seizures. Carbamazepine does not work against absence seizures. It is also approved to treat trigeminal neuralgia. It may cause serious dermatological reactions including toxic epidermal necrolysis (TEN) and Stevens-Johnson Syndrome (SJS) (1 to 6 in 10,000 new patients). It also depresses bone marrow function. Carbamazepine may cause birth defects.

Valproic acid inhibits T-type calcium channels and sodium channels. Valproic acid is used to treat absence seizures and complex partial seizures. Valproic acid should not be used in female patients of childbearing potential because of the serious risks of severe birth defects.

Drugs affecting GABA include barbiturates, benzodiazepines, vigabatrin, and tiagabine. GABA is a natural inhibitor of seizures that works by increasing the flow of Cl^- ion into neurons, which decreases the likelihood of an action potential. Barbiturates and benzodiazepines both increase the amount of chloride ion that flows through $GABA_A$ channels, thus increasing the amount of hyperpolarization, which decreases the likelihood of seizures. Vigabatrin probably decreases the metabolism of GABA by inhibiting GABA transaminase. Tiagabine inhibits the presynaptic reuptake of GABA, similar to how SSRIs work.

Clonazepam is used for absence seizures. Diazepam is used for status epilepticus. Tiagabine is approved for partial seizures. Vigabatrin is approved as adjunctive therapy for refractory complex partial seizures in adults.

Barbiturates and benzodiazepines both cause serious side-effects, including severe CNS depression. Anti-epileptic drugs in general increase suicidal thoughts or behavior. Overdoses of tiagabine have caused seizures and status epilepticus.

Page 64

Anti-epileptic Drugs				
Prolong Sodium Channel Inactivation				
Generic Name / Brand Name	Clinical Use	Dose	Dosage Form	Mechanism of Action
Carbamazepine Tegretol® Epitol®	Partial seizures; generalized tonic clonic seizures, mixed seizure patterns	Adult initial dose: 200 mg twice daily. Maintenance dose: 800-1200 mg daily. Titrate initial dose by 200 mg daily at 7 day intervals.	Generic and Epitol® tablets: 200 mg; generic chewable tablet 100 mg; Tegretol® tablet: 100 mg; oral suspension: 100 mg/5ml 450 ml bottle; generic extended release tablets: 200 mg and 400 mg	Prolongs inactivated state of Na+ channels. This limits the ability of the neuron to fire at high rates, thus reducing the likelihood of an epileptic attack
Lacosamide Vimpat®	Adjunct in the treatment of partial-onset seizures	Adult oral or IV initial dose: 50 mg twice daily, maintenance dose: 200-400 mg/day, titrate by 100 mg/day every 7 days	Vimpat® tablets: 50 mg, 100 mg, 150 mg, and 200 mg; Vimpat® oral solution: 10 mg/ml 20 ml unit dose container; Vimpat® solution for injection: 10 mg/ml 20 ml vial	Enhances slow inactivation of voltage-gated sodium channels
Lamotrigine Lamictal®	Adjunctive in: partial seizures; primary generalized tonic-clonic seizures; generalized seizures of Lennox-Gastaut syndrome; monotherapy for patients older than 16 with partial seizures	Use starter kits for dosing.	Generic and Lamictal® tablets: 25, 100, 150, and 200 mg; Lamictal® ODT orally disintegrating tablets: 25, 50, 100, and 200 mg	Thought to inhibit voltage sensitive sodium channels, thus decreasing a neurons ability to fire, thus decreasing presynaptic release of glutamate and aspartate, two excitatory amino acids
Oxcarbazepine Trileptal®	Monotherapy or adjunct for partial seizures in patients 4 and older; adjunctive therapy for patients 2 and older with partial seizures	Adult monotherapy initial dose: 300 mg twice daily, maintenance dose: 600 mg twice daily, titrate initial dose by 300 mg daily every 3rd day if needed	Generic and Trileptal® tablets: 150 mg, 300 mg, and 600 mg; oral suspension: 300 mg/5ml 250 ml bottle; Trileptal® suspension: 300 mg/5ml 250 ml bottle	Prolongs inactivated state of Na+ channel.

Anti-epileptic Drugs				
Prolong Sodium Channel Inactivation				
Generic Name / Brand Name	Clinical Use	Dose	Dosage Form	Mechanism of Action
Phenytoin Dilantin®	Generalized tonic-clonic seizures; seizure prevention after head trauma or neurosurgery	Adult loading dose of 15 mg to 20 mg/kg. Do not exceed 50 mg per minute. Maintenance doses vary. Usual range 100 mg to 400 mg daily.	Generic extended release capsules: 100, 200, and 300 mg; solution for injection: 50 mg/ml 2ml and 5 ml vials; oral suspension: 125 mg/5ml 120 ml, 237 ml, and 240 ml	Prolongs inactivated state of Na^+ channels. This limits the ability of the neuron to fire at high rates, thus reducing the likelihood of an epileptic attack
Rufinamide Banzel®	Adjunctive treatment of Lennox-Gastaut syndrome	Adult initial dose: 400-800 mg/day in 2 divided doses, maintenance dose: 3200 mg/day in 2 equal doses. Titrate by 400-800 mg every other day until 3200 mg daily or 45 mg/kg/day, whichever is less, is reached.	Banzel® tablets: 200 mg and 400 mg; Banzel® oral suspension: 40 mg/ml 460 ml bottle	Extends the inactive state of voltage-gated sodium channels, thus decreasing repetitive firings or depolarizations. May inhibit excitatory glutamate receptors (mGluR5).
Topiramate Topamax®	Monotherapy for epilepsy. Adjunctive therapy for epilepsy. Prophylaxis of migraine headache.	Initial adult monotherapy dose 25 mg BID. Recommended maintenance dose of 200 mg BID.	Generic and Topamax® tablets: 25mg, 50 mg, 100 mg, and 200 mg	Blocks voltage-dependent Na^+ channels. Augments GABA at $GABA_A$ receptors. Inhibits the AMPA/kainate subtype of glutamate receptors. Inhibits carbonic anhydrase enzyme
Valproic Acid Depakene®	Monotherapy or adjunctive therapy of complex partial seizures, and simple and complex absence seizures	Adult initial dose 10 mg to 15 mg/kg/day. Best response obtained at dose lower than 60 mg/kg/day.	Generic and Depakene® capsules: 250 mg; generic solution for injection: 100 mg/ml 5ml vials; generic and Depakene® oral solution: 250 mg/5ml 5ml unit dose containers and 473 ml bottles	Prolongs inactivated state of Na^+ channels. Reduces T-type Ca^{2+} currents
Zonisamide Zonegran®	Adjunctive therapy of partial seizures in patients 16 and older	Initial dose: 100 mg daily. Usual maintenance dose: 100-200 mg daily. Titrate dose by 100 mg daily every 14 days, max dose: 400 mg daily	Capsules 100 mg and 200 mg	Prolongs the inactivated state of voltage-gated Na^+ channels. Reduces T-type Ca^{2+} currents.

Anti-Epileptic Drugs Inhibition of T-type Calcium Channels (Located in nerve cell body)				
Generic Name / Brand Name	Use	Dose	Dosage Form	Mechanism of Action
Ethosuximide Zarontin®	Absence seizures	Adult initial oral dose: 500 mg once daily. Must individualize dose per patient.	Generic and Zarontin® capsules: 250 mg; generic and Zarontin® oral solution: 250 mg/5ml 473 ml and 480 ml bottles respectively	Reduces T-type low-threshold Ca^{2+} currents
Valproic Acid Depakene®	Monotherapy or adjunctive treatment of complex partial seizures, and simple and complex absence seizures	Adult initial dose 10 mg to 15 mg/kg/day. Best response obtained at dose lower than 60 mg/kg/day.	Generic and Depakene® capsules: 250 mg; generic solution for injection: 100 mg/ml 5ml vials; generic and Depakene® oral solution: 250 mg/5ml 5ml unit dose containers and 473 ml bottles	Reduces T-type Ca^{2+} currents. Prolongs inactivated state of Na^+ channels.
Zonisamide Zonegran®	Adjunctive therapy of partial seizures in patients 16 and older	Initial dose: 100 mg daily, maintenance dose: 100-400 mg daily, titrate dose by 100 mg daily every 14 days, max dose: 400 mg daily	Capsules 100 mg and 200 mg	Reduces T-type Ca^{2+} currents.
Inhibition of High-Voltage-Activated Calcium Channels (located at presynaptic nerve ending)				
Gabapentin Neurontin®	Adjunct for partial seizures, with or without secondary generalization	Starting dose of 300 mg three times daily. This may be too tiring for some patients; may need to start at a lower dose. Maintenance dose of 900 mg to 1800 mg daily.	Generic and Neurontin® capsules: 100 mg, 300 mg, and 400 mg; generic and Gabapentin oral solution: 250 mg/5ml 470 ml bottle; generic tablets: 600 mg and 800 mg	Mechanism of action is unclear; binds to alpha$_2$-delta-1 subunit of HVA calcium channels, thereby decreasing release of excitatory neurotransmitters
Pregabalin Lyrica®	Adjunctive treatment for adult patients with partial onset seizures	Adult initial oral dose: 50 mg three times daily, maintenance dose: 150-600 mg daily, titrate based on side-effects, max dose: 600 mg daily	Lyrica® capsules: 25 mg, 50 mg, 75 mg, 100 mg, 150 mg, 200 mg, 225 mg, and 300 mg	Mechanism of action is unclear; binds to alpha$_2$-delta-1 HVA calcium channels, thereby decreasing release of excitatory neurotransmitters.

GABA Reuptake Inhibitors and GABA-T Inhibitors

Generic Name / Brand Name	Use	Dose	Dosage Form	Mechanism of Action
Tiagabine Gabitril®	Adjunct therapy for patients 12 and older with partial seizures	Adult patients already on CYP inducing drugs: initial oral dose: 4 mg daily, maintenance dose: 32-56 mg daily in divided doses. Titrate by 4-8 mg every 7 days. For patients not on CYP inducing drugs the dose must be lowered.	Gabitril® tablets: 2 mg, 4 mg, 12 mg, and 16 mg	Prevents the presynaptic re-uptake of GABA by inhibiting GAT-1 (GABA transporter).
Vigabatrin Sabril®	Sabril® Oral Solution treats Infantile Spasms (IS); Tablets are adjunctive therapy for Refractory Complex Partial Seizures in Adults	Adult initial oral dose: 500 mg twice daily, Recommended maintenance dose: 1.5 grams twice daily. Titrate by 500 mg daily every 7 days, max dose: 3000 mg daily	Sabril® tablets: 500 mg	Thought to inhibit GABA-Transaminase, the enzyme that metabolizes GABA

Synaptic Vesicle Protein (SV2A)

Generic Name / Brand Name	Use	Dose	Dosage Form	Mechanism of Action
Levetiracetam Keppra® Keppra® XR	Adjunctive therapy for partial onset, myoclonic, and primary generalized tonic-clonic seizures	Adult initial oral dose for partial onset seizure: 500 mg twice daily. If maintenance dose: 1000-3000 mg daily in divided dose, max dose: 3 grams daily. Titrate by 500 mg BID every two weeks if needed.	Generic tablets: 250 mg, 500 mg, 750 mg, and 1000 mg; Keppra® tablets: 250 mg, 500 mg, and 750 mg; generic and Keppra® extended release tablets: 500 mg and 750 mg; generic oral solution: 100 mg/ml 5 ml unit-dose and 480 ml bottles; Keppra® oral solution 100 mg/ml 480 ml bottle.	Interaction with SV2A, a synaptic vesicle protein, thought to be MOA

Page 68

CHAPTER 9

HYPNOTICS AND SEDATIVES

Benzodiazepines		Barbiturates	"Z" Compounds
Alprazolam Chlordiazepoxide Clonazepam Clorazepate Diazepam Estazolam Flurazepam	Lorazepam Midazolam Oxazepam Quazepam Temazepam Triazolam	Amobarbital Pentobarbital Phenobarbital Methohexital Secobarbital	Eszopiclone Zaleplon Zolpidem

All three classes are agonists at the gamma-aminobutyric acid (GABA$_A$) receptor. GABA is the major inhibitory neurotransmitter in the central nervous system. As agonists, benzodiazepines and barbiturates depress the CNS along a continuum. At low doses they are anxiolytics, muscle relaxants, sedatives, and hypnotics. At higher doses they both induce anesthesia. At higher doses barbiturates cause medullary depression (decreased respiration). Finally, barbiturates, even when given alone, can cause coma and death at high enough doses. In contrast, benzodiazepines alone do not cause death at high doses; however, administering alcohol or other sedative drugs with benzodiazepines at high doses can cause death. The "Z" compounds are the newest members of the group. They are used solely to treat insomnia. Benzodiazepines and barbiturates have distinct binding sites on the GABA$_A$ receptor. Z compounds and benzodiazepines have overlapping binding sites on the GABA$_A$ receptor. Baclofen is the only marketed drug that binds with GABA$_B$ receptors; its treats muscle spasms for patients with MS. Baclofen is also an agonist.

Hypnotic drugs cause sleep. Sedative drugs cause sedation. Barbiturates and benzodiazepines are "sedative-hypnotics" because they cause sedation at low doses and sleep at higher doses. Clinicians used barbiturates for several decades as sedative-hypnotics. Serious side-effects, including death, led to the development of benzodiazepines. Today, benzodiazepines are the primary sedative-hypnotics; however, some barbiturates are still used for specific purposes such as intubating patients before surgery. The newest class of hypnotics is referred to as the "Z" compounds, which are non-benzodiazepine hypnotics. Zolpidem is perhaps the most well known example. Just as benzodiazepines improved upon barbiturates by decreasing the possibility of severe respiratory depression, the "Z" compounds exhibit less side-effects than benzodiazepines; in particular, they cause less falls.

BENZODIAZEPINES

Benzodiazepines can be used as anxiolytics, sedatives, hypnotics, muscle relaxants, and anticonvulsants. Some are also used for amnestic effects. Midazolam and diazepam are used to induce anesthesia. Diazepam, lorazepam, clonazepam, and clorazepate treat seizures. Clorazepate is FDA approved as an adjunctive therapy to treat focal seizures (partial seizures).

Benzodiazepines work by binding with GABA$_A$ receptors in the brain. When benzodiazepines bind to GABA$_A$ receptors, they facilitate the binding of gamma-aminobutyric acid (GABA) to GABA$_A$ receptors. GABA is one of the principal inhibitory neurotransmitters of the brain. Consequently, drugs promoting the binding of GABA to GABA$_A$ receptors inhibit brain functions. Benzodiazepines increase the frequency at which the chloride ion channel opens, which allows more Cl$^-$ ion than normal to enter the cell making it more polarized, and thus unable to initiate an action potential. GABA binds with three different receptors: GABA$_A$, GABA$_B$, and GABA$_C$. Baclofen is the only marketed drug that affects GABA$_B$ receptors. There are no marketed drugs available that bind with GABA$_C$ receptors. The barbiturates and benzodiazepines have distinct binding sites.

Usually benzodiazepines are not drugs of choice for treating epilepsy because of their severe side-effects such as drowsiness, ataxia, and dizziness.

However, intravenous diazepam and lorazepam are drugs of choice for treating status epilepticus. Diazepam can also be administered rectally to treat status epilepticus. Diazepam is not generally used for long-term management of seizures because it causes too much day-time sedation. In contrast, clonazepam and clorazepate are approved for the long-term treatment of seizures; however, they are generally not first line drugs.

DRUG INTERACTIONS

CYP3A4 metabolizes most benzodiazepines. Inhibitors of CYP3A4, such as clarithromycin, erythromycin, grapefruit juice, itraconazole, ketoconazole, nefazodone, and others can significantly increase blood levels of benzodiazepines. After metabolism by CYP3A4, some benzodiazepines are further metabolized to glucuronides. Inducers of CYP3A4, such as nifedipine, omeprazole, and rifampin, may decrease blood levels of benzodiazepines. Benzodiazepines themselves do not induce or inhibit CYP isoenzymes.

Z COMPOUNDS

Zolpidem and zaleplon are FDA approved for the short-term treatment of insomnia. Eszopiclone is approved for the long-term treatment of insomnia. The Z compounds lack anxiolytic and muscle relaxant properties.

Zolpidem, eszopiclone, and zaleplon, preferentially bind with $GABA_A$ receptors that only have the $alpha_1$ subunit. All of the "Z-compounds" or "Z-drugs" bind with $GABA_A$ receptors close to the site where benzodiazepines bind, if not actually overlapping.

Zolpidem, eszopiclone, and zaleplon each shorten sleep latency. Z compounds generally start working within 30 minutes of administration.

Absorption is rapid and nearly complete for all three drugs. Large volume of distributions characterize each drug, reflecting their lipophilic nature.

CYP3A4 metabolizes each to various extents. Ketoconazole, a strong inhibitor of CYP3A4, increases zolpidem's levels substantially, a dose reduction may be necessary. Ketoconazole also substantially increases levels of eszopiclone; the starting dose of eszopiclone should be 1mg when coadministered with a potent CYP3A4 inhibitor such as itraconazole, clarithromycin, nefazodone, troleandomycin, ritonavir, and nelfinavir. Zaleplon is primarily metabolized by aldehyde oxidase,

and only slightly by CYP3A4; all of its metabolites are inactive.

BARBITURATES

Barbiturates are used for seizures, preanesthetics, anxiety before surgery, and rarely as sedative-hypnotics. Phenobarbital is used to treat tonic-clonic (grand mal) seizures, status epilepticus, and focal seizures (partial seizures). It is also approved as a sedative-hypnotic, however, because much safer sedative-hypnotics are available, it is rarely used for insomnia. Amobarbital is FDA approved to treat anxiety prior to surgery and produce sedation prior to surgery. It is also approved as a hypnotic for the short-term treatment of insomnia. Pentobarbital is FDA approved to treat status epilepticus and as a sedative-hypnotic. Secobarbital is approved FDA approved for the short-term treatment of insomnia and as a preanesthetic. Methohexital is FDA approved to induce anesthesia.

Barbiturates have several mechanisms of action: 1) promote the binding of GABA to $GABA_A$ receptors, 2) at high concentrations, they activate $GABA_A$ receptors even without GABA being present, and 3) inhibit AMPA receptors (usually activated by the excitatory neurotransmitter glutamate). The second mechanism of action accounts for the fact that barbiturates cause medullary depression, coma, and death.

Barbiturates increase the time the $GABA_A$ receptor remains open, thus allowing more chloride ion to pass into the neuron, hyperpolarizing it, and, finally, therefore, unlikely to conduct an action potential. Chloride ion, being negatively charged, increases the relative difference between the amount of overall negative charge inside a neuron and the overall amount of positive charge outside of a neuron.

The barbiturate site is located in the middle of the receptor. The area where GABA binds is distinct from where the barbiturates and benzodiazepines bind.

A barbiturate's onset of action depends on its lipophilicity. The greater the lipophilicity, the faster the onset of action. Thiopental and methohexital, being the most lipophilic, work the fastest, usually in 10 to 30 seconds, after IV administration. Pentobarbital works in a minute or less after IV administration; and upto an hour after oral administration. In contrast, phenobarbital, being much less lipophilic, works about 5 minutes after IV administration. Secobarbital, only administered orally, may take an hour to sedate a patient before surgery.

Phenobarbital and primidone are the two main barbiturates used today as anticonvulsants. Phenobarbital treats focal (partial) seizures and generalized tonic-clonic seizures. Primidone treats focal seizures, psychomotor seizures, and generalized tonic-clonic seizures. Phenobarbital is dosed at 100 mg to 200 mg daily. Primidone is dosed at 750 mg to 1000 mg in three divided doses because of its shorter-half. Phenobarbital and primidone both cause drowsiness, nystagmus (eye twitching), and ataxia, among other side-effects.

Phenobarbital, the main barbiturate still used in outpatient treatment, is about 25% excreted unchanged by the kidneys. The other 75% is metabolized by CYP2C9. Phenobarbital induces CYP2C and CYP3A-subfamilies of isoenzymes. This can interfere with oral contraceptives which are metabolized by CYP3A4. Further, phenobarbital induces UGT enzymes.

Benzodiazepines				
Generic Name / Brand Name	Clinical Use	Dose	Half Life	Dosage Form
Alprazolam Xanax® Xanax® XR	Generalized anxiety disorder (GAD); panic disorder; agoraphobia	Adult dose for anxiety disorders: 0.25 mg to 0.5 mg three times daily.	12 hours	Generic and Xanax® tablets: 0.25, 0.5, 1, and 2 mg; Alprazolam Intensol oral solution: 1 mg/ml 30 ml bottle; generic orally disintegrating tablet: 0.25, 0.5, 1, and 2 mg
Chlordiazepoxide Librium®	Anxiety, withdrawal from alcohol	Adult initial dose 5 mg once daily. Maintenance dose 5 mg to 10 mg 3 to 4 times daily.	10 hours	Generic capsules: 5, 10, and 25 mg
Clonazepam Klonopin®	Panic disorders; seizures	Adult oral dose for panic disorder: 0.25 mg twice daily for 3 days. Recommended maintenance dose of 1 mg daily.	23 hours	Generic and Klonopin® tablets: 0.5, 1, and 2 mg; orally disintegrating tablets: 0.125, 0.25, 0.5, 1, and 2 mg
Clorazepate Tranxene®	GAD; alcohol withdrawal; adjunct to treatment of partial seizures	Adult dose for GAD: 7.5-15 mg two to four times daily	2 hours	Generic and Tranxene® tablets: 3.75, 7.5, and 15 mg
Diazepam Valium®	Anxiety, alcohol withdrawal, skeletal muscle relaxant, convulsive disorders	Adult oral, IM, or IV dose for anxiety: 2 mg 2 to 4 times daily, may increase to 10 mg four times daily as needed	43 hours	Generic and Valium® tablets: 2, 5, and 10 mg
Estazolam Prosom®	Insomnia	Adult dose: 0.5 mg at bedtime, maintenance dose: 0.5-2 mg at bedtime	10-24 hours	Generic tablets: 1 and 2 mg
Flurazepam Dalmane	Insomnia	Adult dose: 15-30 mg at bedtime	74 hours	Generic capsules: 15 and 30 mg
Lorazepam Ativan®	Anxiety; insomnia	Adult dose: 0.5-2mg twice daily, max dose of 10 mg daily	14 hours	Generic and Ativan® tablets: 0.5, 1, and 2 mg
Midazolam Versed	Preanesthetic; maintenance of anesthesia	Adult IV dose: 0.02-0.04 mg/kg, may repeat every five minutes as needed upto 4 times, total max dose of 0.1-0.2 mg/kg	2 hours	Solution for injection: 1 mg/ml 2 ml, 5 ml, and 10 ml vials, 5 mg/ml 1 ml, 2 ml, 5 ml, and 10 ml vials; oral syrup: 2 mg/ml 118 ml bottle

Benzodiazepines				
Generic Name / Brand Name	Clinical Use	Dose	Half Life	Dosage Form
Oxazepam Serax	Anxiety; alcohol withdrawal	Adult oral dose for anxiety: 10-30 mg 3 to 4 times daily	8 hours	Generic capsules: 10, 15, and 30 mg
Quazepam Doral	Insomnia	Adult oral initial dose: 15 mg at bedtime, maintenance dose: 7.5-15 mg at bedtime	39 hours	Generic tablet: 15 mg
Temazepam Restoril®	Insomnia	Adult dose: 7.5-30 mg at bedtime	11 hours	Generic and Restoril® capsules: 7.5, 15, 22.5, and 30 mg
Triazolam Halcion®	Insomnia	Adult dose: 0.125-0.25 mg at bedtime, maintenance dose: 0.125-0.5 mg at bedtime, max dose of 0.5mg	3 hours	Generic tablet: 0.125 and 0.25 mg; Halcion® tablets: 0.25

Barbiturates				
Generic Name Brand Name	Clinical Use	Dose	Mechanism of Action	Dosage Form
Amobarbital Amytal®	Hypnotic for insomnia; anxiolytic and sedative for preop	Adult hypnotic IM or IV dose: 65-200 mg at bedtime, max dose of 1000 mg	Promotes the binding of GABA to its receptor $GABA_A$	Powder for reconstitution for injection: 500 mg vials
Methohexital Brevital®	Induction of anesthesia	Adult dose 1-1.5 mg/kg	Same as above	Powder for reconstitution for injection: 500 mg vial and 2.5 gram vial
Pentobarbital Nembutal®	Sedative; hypnotic; refractory status epilepticus	Adult hypnotic and sedative IV, initial dose: 100 mg, may repeat dose with at least one minute intervals, max total dose of 500 mg	Same as above	Nembutal® solution for injection: 50 mg/ml 20 ml and 50 ml vials
Phenobarbital	Generalized tonic-clonic (grand mal) seizures; status epilepticus, and partial seizures;	Adult anticonvulsant maintenance oral dose: 50-100 mg 2 to 3 times daily	Same as above	Tablets: 15, 30, 60, and 100 mg
Secobarbital Seconal®	Preanesthesia; short-term treatment of insomnia	Adult sedation for surgery oral dose: 100-300 mg 1 to 2 hours before	Same as above	Seconal® capsule: 100 mg

CHAPTER 10

LOCAL ANESTHETICS

Local anesthetics cause anesthesia in an area limited to the site of administration or areas close by or areas controlled by spinal nerves that have been blocked, as opposed, to general anesthetics which cause loss of sensation throughout the body. Patients can remain awake with local anesthetics. Local anesthetics are used for infiltration anesthesia or nerve block anesthesia. Infiltration anesthesia is used for when a small area needs to be anesthetized such as dental procedures. When larger areas need to be anesthetized, nerve block anesthesia (regional anesthesia) is used. Nerve block anesthesia includes many different types of anesthesia including spinal anesthesia and epidural anesthesia. Preservative free anesthetics must be used for these procedures.

All local anesthetics have the same mechanism of action, they block sodium channels in nerves preventing transmission of nerve impulses. Nerve impulses depend, in part, on sodium ions flowing from the exterior of a neuron through voltage gated sodium ion channels to the interior of a neuron. Local anesthetics work by physically blocking, from inside the neuron, voltage gated sodium ion channels thus preventing sodium ions from passing through the ion channels. Blocking of neuronal sodium ion channels prevents the conduction of nerve impulses to the CNS and from the CNS.

Traditionally, local anesthetics are divided into two classes based on their chemical structure. Anesthetics with a ester group include cocaine, benzocaine procaine, and tetracaine. Anesthetics with an amide group include lidocaine, bupivacaine, mepivacaine, prilocaine, ropivacaine, and dibucaine. Interestingly, cocaine was the first used anesthetic; however, its addictive properties were quickly recognized, prompting the search for other drugs.

As an overall group, local anesthetics have the same general pattern for their chemical structures. The aforementioned ester groups and amide groups function as a bridge between a hydrophobic aromatic ring on one end of the drug and a secondary or tertiary amine group on the opposite end, which is hydrophilic. Both ester and amide anesthetics have the same mechanism of action. Their structures cause them to differ in their duration of action. Plasma esterases, which are metabolizing enzymes found in the blood, quickly and easily metabolize anesthetics with an ester group. In contrast, amide anesthetics are metabolized by the CYP450 system in the liver. Amide anesthetics have a substantially longer duration of action because they have to be absorbed into the blood stream and delivered to the liver before they can be inactivated.

Because local anesthetics are systemically absorbed from their site of application, they can cause severe side-effects. Local anesthetics can affect sodium channels in the brain, heart, lungs, intestinal tract, and other areas. These side-effects can be severe and life-threatening. Central nervous system side-effects include drowsiness, confusion, convulsions, initial excitation of the CNS and then CNS depression. Local anesthetics can depress neurons controlling respiration, leading to respiratory depression or respiratory arrest. Further, local anesthetics can affect the heart. They can reduce conduction velocity and cardiac contractility. Bupivacaine, at high doses, can generate arrhythmias.

Lidocaine works quickly and lasts between one to two hours; as with all drugs, lidocaine's chemical structure influences its duration of action. As a relatively hydrophobic molecule, it stays in neurons longer; further, its amide bond prevents metabolism by plasma esterases. Lidocaine is available in a patch formulation that lasts for 12 hours. It is also available as a gel and injection.

Lidocaine and prilocaine are available as a combination product called EMLA®. EMLA is approved for local analgesia and for application to genital mucous membranes. The dose is highly individualized. As a starting dose, use one to two grams per 10 cm². The manufacturer recommends applying EMLA one hour before venipuncture and two hours before skin grafts. EMLA should not be used in patients who have methemoglobinemia.

Tetracaine is used for both local anesthesia and spinal anesthesia. Tetracaine has a rapid onset of action. Tetracaine lasts for two to three hours. Tetracaine has a long duration of action because of the large four (hence "tetra") carbon chain on the aromatic ring. This four carbon chain increases its hydrophobicity, allowing it to stay in neurons longer than other ester anesthetics.

Procaine is typically used as an infiltration anesthetic and for dental procedures. It can be used for diagnostic nerve blocks. It has a fast onset of action and short duration of action.

Bupivacaine is a long acting amide anesthetic. It is indicated for local or regional anesthesia for surgery, dental procedures, diagnostic procedures, and obstetrical procedures. Always give in small test doses with enough time between doses to monitor for adverse effects, particularly cardiac effects in obstetrical patients.

Local Anesthetics				
Generic Name / Brand Name	Clinical Use	Mechanism of Action	Adverse Effects	Contraindications
Amides				
Bupivacaine Marcaine®	Local and regional anesthesia. Obstetrical procedures. Dental and oral surgery.	Blocks Na^+ channel in neuronal membranes, preventing the nerve from generating an action potential.	CNS excitation or CNS depression resulting from excessive dose reaching systemic circulation. Cardiac arrest usually from excessively high doses reaching systemic circulation	Known sensitivity to amide anesthetics, infection at site of administration
Lidocaine Xylocaine®	Local or regional anesthesia, short-term treatment of ventricular arrhythmias caused by myocardial infarction or cardiac manipulation	Same as above	Same as above	Same as above
Mepivacaine Carbocaine®	Local or regional anesthesia, anesthesia by peripheral and central neural administration	Same as above	Same as above	Same as above
Ropivacaine Naropin®	Anesthetic for surgery, pain after surgery	Same as above	Same as above	Same as above
Esters				
Chloroprocaine Nesacaine®, Nesacaine®-MPF	Infiltration anesthesia, epidural, peripheral nerve block	Same as above	CNS excitation or depression. Toxic blood levels decrease cardiac conduction and excitability, possible cardiac arrest	For lumbar and caudal epidural anesthesia use extreme caution in patients with existing neurological disease, spinal deformities, septicemia, and severe hypertension. Infection at site of administration.
Tetracaine Pontocaine®	Spinal or topical anesthesia	Same as above	Same as above	Infection as site of administration

CHAPTER 11

CARDIOVASCULAR DRUGS

Alpha Blockers	Beta Blockers	Calcium Channel Blockers	Renin Angiotensin System	Diuretics
Non-Selective Alpha$_1$ and alpha$_2$ blockers: Phenoxybenzamine Phentolamine **Non-Selective Alpha$_1$ blockers:** Prazosin Terazosin Doxazosin	**Non-Selective:** Propranolol Labetalol **Selective:** Atenolol Metoprolol	**Dihydropyridines:** Amlodipine Nifedipine Isradipine Felodipine **Non-Dihydropyridines:** Diltiazem Verapamil	**Direct Renin Inhibitors:** Aliskiren **ACE Inhibitors:** Lisinopril Quinapril Ramipril **ARBs:** Losartan Valsartan Olmesartan	**Loop:** Furosemide Torsemide Bumetanide **Thiazide:** Hydrochlorothiazide Chlorothiazide **K$^+$ Sparing:** Spironolactone Triamterene

Thiazide diuretics are considered the best first choice for patients with hypertension because overall they produce better cardiovascular outcomes and have fewer side-effects than other antihypertensive drugs. However, at least two-thirds of patients eventually require two or more antihypertensive drugs. Thiazide diuretics can be combined with any of the other antihypertensives.

The older non-selective alpha-blockers are primarily used in hospitalized patients. However they are used on an out-patient basis for patients who are waiting for surgery to treat pheochromocytoma. The newer selective beta-blockers are preferred over the older, non-selective beta-blockers because they do not affect the lungs. The dihydropyridines are better at treating hypertension than the non-dihydropyridines. However, the non-dihydropyridines are used to treat arrhythmias.

Losartan is particularly beneficial at treating hypertension and reducing mortality.

Many drugs treat hypertension (high blood pressure), angina (a lack of oxygen to the heart causing pain), heart failure, and arrhythmias. These drugs include alpha blockers, ACE inhibitors, angiotensin receptor blockers (ARBs), renin inhibitors, beta blockers, cardiac glycosides, diuretics, and direct vasodilators. For most cases of hypertension, the cause is unknown; this is called essential hypertension. Some cases of hypertension are secondary to another disease state.

ALPHA BLOCKERS

Alpha blockers prevent norepinephrine and epinephrine (catecholamines) from binding with alpha receptors, located in arteries and veins, thus stopping the increase in blood pressure that would otherwise occur. Alpha blockers have two main classes: 1) non-selective (block alpha$_1$ and alpha$_2$; and 2) alpha$_1$ selective.

Alpha$_1$ selective blockers are also further subdivided based on their affinities for the various alpha$_1$ receptor subtypes, see below and table at end of chapter. The non-selective alpha blockers phentolamine and phenoxybenzamine treat pheochromocytoma. Phentolamine is used to diagnose pheochromocytoma.

The alpha$_1$ selective blockers, terazosin, doxazosin, and prazosin treat hypertension. Alpha$_1$ blockers also treat benign prostatic hyperplasia (BPH) by decreasing the pressure the prostate applies to the bladder neck, allowing for easier urination.

Alfuzosin, tamsulosin, and silodosin are also alpha$_1$ selective antagonists; however, they are approved to treat benign prostatic hypertrophy (BPH), not hypertension. Alfuzosin is a selective antagonist at postsynaptic alpha$_1$ receptors. Blocking these receptors relaxes smooth muscle in the bladder neck and prostate, easing urination.

Alpha blockers should not be used alone to treat hypertension. Rather, they are usually used in various combinations with beta-blockers, diuretics, and other antihypertensives.

In contrast to alpha blockers acting outside of the CNS, clonidine acts in the CNS as an alpha$_2$ agonist. Clonidine decreases blood pressure by acting as an agonist at alpha$_2$ receptors. Alpha$_2$ receptors are located on presynaptic neurons in the CNS. Activation of alpha$_2$ receptors decreases sympathetic outflow, which decreases blood pressure. Activating alpha$_2$ receptors tells the neuron that it has released enough sympathetic outflow (norepinephrine), and, therefore, needs to stop releasing norepinephrine onto the postsynaptic neuron.

SIDE-EFFECTS

Alpha blockers can cause orthostatic hypotension. Administer them at bedtime because of this side-effect. Doxazosin, terazosin, and prazosin should be administered at bedtime so if postural hypotension occurs, the patient will be asleep thus eliminating any chance of falling down.

DRUG INTERACTIONS

Alpha blockers can potentiate or increase the effects of other antihypertensive drugs, potentially decreasing blood pressure too much, which may lead to falls in elderly patients. Alfuzosin can prolong the heart's QT interval, and, therefore, should not be given to patients who have QT prolongation or at risk for it. Further, it should no be administered with CYP3A4 inhibitors because they will increase blood levels of alfuzosin.

BETA BLOCKERS

Beta blockers treat glaucoma (timolol), hypertension, angina pectoris, left ventricular dysfunction after myocardial infarction, congestive heart failure, ischemic heart disease, and some arrhythmias. Beta blockers decrease heart rate (negative chronotropic effect), decrease cardiac contractility (negative inotropic effect), decrease blood pressure, and decrease the heart's demand for oxygen. Also, long-term use of beta blockers causes total peripheral resistance to decrease in patients with hypertension.

Beta blockers are traditionally classified as 1) non-selective and 2) beta$_1$ selective antagonists. The

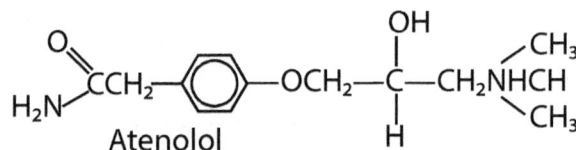
Atenolol

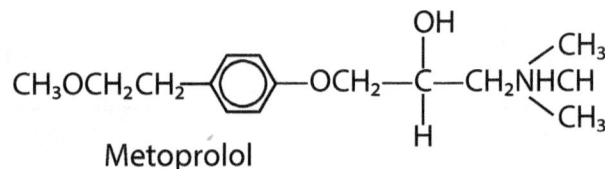
Metoprolol

desire to selectively inhibit beta$_1$ versus beta$_2$ receptors stems from the fact that beta$_2$ receptors are found in the lungs. Antagonism or blockade of these receptors can cause breathing difficulties, and in asthmatics, has been fatal. Carvedilol and labetalol block both beta receptors and alpha$_1$ receptors. Despite blocking both beta receptors, carvedilol is frequently used because of its superior cardiovascular benefits. Further, carvedilol actually improves the body's ability to use insulin in patients with insulin resistance.

The two most commonly used selective beta$_1$ blockers are metoprolol and atenolol. You can see from the structures of each, that atenolol and metoprolol are quite similar. However, the structures are different enough to alter the pharmacokinetics of each. Metoprolol is usually dosed twice daily and atenolol is usually dosed once daily.

Propranolol, a non-selective beta blocker, treats migraine headaches, angina pectoris, hypertrophic subaortic stenosis, and hypertension. It is contraindicated in patients with cardiogenic shock, sinus bradycardia, and bronchial asthma. Do not stop propranolol without slowing tapering the dose because that can cause myocardial infarction or aggravate angina pectoris. Because it has a short duration of action, it is available in long acting formulations. As a generic medication, it is relatively inexpensive.

SIDE-EFFECTS

Older and non-selective beta-blockers can cause bronchioles to constrict in asthmatics, causing difficulty breathing. In addition, beta blockers complicate diabetes in two main ways. Beta-blockers can mask the signs of hypoglycemia such as increased heart rate and tremor. Second, non-selective beta blockers may prevent the conversion of glycogen to glucose, thus preventing recovery from low blood sugar (hypoglycemia); beta$_1$ selective blockers inhibit recovery much less than the non-selective blockers. Further, the older beta blockers (propranolol) decrease sensitivity to insulin, meaning the body needs more insulin to move glucose from the bloodstream into cells.

DRUG INTERACTIONS

Beta blockers, when combined with other anti-hypertensives, may lower blood pressure too much; care must be used when administering multiple anti-hypertensives. Beta blockers can interfere with antidiabetic drugs by masking the signs of hypoglycemia. A patient may not realize he or she needs to skip a dose of antidiabetic medication because his or her blood sugar is too low and the signs are masked by a beta blocker.

RENIN ANGIOTENSIN SYSTEM

The renin angiotensin system (RAS) raises blood pressure in times of cardiovascular shock. However, this system can be activated even when the body is not in cardiovascular shock, thus leading to hypertension. Angiotensin II is the end product of the RAS that actually raises blood pressure. To make angiotensin II, the body starts with angiotensinogen, which it converts (with an enzyme called renin) to an intermediary called angiotensin I. Angiotensin I gets converted to angiotensin II by an enzyme called angiotensin converting enzyme (ACE). Angiotensin II raises blood pressure by binding with the angiotensin receptor called AT-1. Angiotensin I, relative to angiotensin II, only slightly raises blood pressure.

Three types of drugs decrease blood pressure by blocking the renin angiotensin system: 1) direct renin inhibitors, 2) angiotensin converting enzyme inhibitors, and 3) angiotensin receptor blockers. Direct renin inhibitors block the enzyme renin from converting angiotensinogen to angiotensin I. Angiotensin converting enzyme inhibitors block the conversion of angiotensin I to angiotensin II. Angiotensin receptor (AT-1) blockers (ARBs) prevent angiotensin II from binding with the AT-1 receptor. ARBs are more effective than ACE inhibitors at preventing the activation of AT-1 receptors. Angiotensin II can be formed by alternative pathways that do not require ACE, and thus, in the absence of an ARB, it can still stimulate AT-1 receptors. In addition to lowering blood pressure, losartan is indicated for diabetic nephropathy and stroke prevention. Irbesartan is also indicated for diabetic nephropathy. Valsartan is indicated for heart failure and to reduce mortality in patients with left ventricular dysfunction following a myocardial infarction. ARBs protect the kidneys in

patients who have type II diabetes mellitus. Aliskiren is a direct renin inhibitor.

SIDE-EFFECTS

Overall, ACE inhibitors are well tolerated. ACE inhibitors can cause cough and angioedema. ACE inhibitors may cause hyperkalemia in diabetic patients and in patients with poorly functioning kidneys. Aliskiren is well tolerated in most patients, including those with decreased renal function and hepatic disease. Aliskiren causes mild gastrointestinal problems, including gastroesophageal reflux disease. Aliskiren causes less cough problems than ACE inhibitors.

DRUG INTERACTIONS

ACE inhibitors combined with potassium supplements or beta-blockers may lead to excess potassium in the blood (hyperkalemia). ACE inhibitors can also increase digoxin levels. NSAIDS and aspirin may reduce the effectiveness of ACE inhibitors.

ARBs may cause hyperkalemia in patients taking potassium supplements or potassium sparing diuretics; hyperkalemia has also occurred in patients with renal disease.

Administration of aliskiren with fatty foods decreases the absorption of aliskiren. P-gp, a pump that prevents certain drugs from being absorbed, substantially decreases the absorption of aliskiren. However, inhibitors of P-gp increase blood levels of aliskiren. Some P-gp inhibitors are atorvastatin, cyclosporine, and ketoconazole.

DIURETICS

Excess fluid volume may cause hypertension and exacerbate heart failure. The removal of this extra fluid reduces blood pressure and may ameliorate heart failure.

The body must keep electrolytes (sodium, potassium, chloride, and calcium) within certain ranges to maintain life. The kidneys are responsible for keeping these electrolytes within these ranges. Nephrons, the functional units of kidneys, are tubes starting at arterioles (small arteries) and ending at collecting ducts that drain urine. The major parts of a nephron are the Bowman's capsule, glomerulus, proximal tubule, descending loop of Henle, ascending loop of Henle, proximal convoluted tubule, distal convoluted tubule, and collecting duct.

The Bowman's capsule is the beginning of a nephron. The Bowman's capsule forms a cup-shaped structure. Inside the Bowman's capsule is the glomerulus. The glomerulus is a set of capillaries derived from an arteriole. Plasma flows into these capillaries. Small particles pass from the capillaries and into the Bowman's capsule to begin their journey through the nephron. Proteins stay in the blood and return to the general circulation.

The fluid and solutes that filter into the glomerulus is called "filtrate." Hence, the first step in urine formation is called "filtration." "Reabsorption," the opposite of "filtration," is the passage of electrolytes and/or water from inside the nephron ultimately back into the blood. "Secretion," another aspect of urine formation, is the passage of electrolytes from the space between nephrons (interstitial fluid) back into the nephron to be excreted. "Excretion" is the movement of fluid and electrolytes into the urine. A water molecule that is filtered at the glomerulus and never reabsorbed is said to be "excreted." Similarly, a potassium ion that is "secreted" from interstitial fluid into the tubules and not "reabsorbed" is said to be "excreted."

Characteristics of the nephron combined with characteristics of the various areas of the interstitial fluid allow the body to precisely control how much water and electrolytes are removed from the body. For conceptual purposes, think of the interstitial fluid as having several layers that differ in tonicity (how much solutes are dissolved in a fluid). Nephrons pass through these layers differing in tonicity. Some parts of the nephron allow water to easily pass through it; some parts of the nephron do not allow water to pass through it. Further, some parts of the nephron allow specific electrolytes to pass out of it, and some areas of the nephron allow electrolytes to move into it (secretion), and some parts of the nephron do not allow electrolytes to move in, nor, out of it.

LOOP DIURETICS

Loop diuretics include furosemide, bumetanide, ethacrynic acid, and torsemide. Loop diuretics work in the thick ascending part of the loop of Henle. They stop the sodium-potassium-chloride pump from reabsorbing sodium and chloride, further they increase the amount of potassium excreted in the urine, meaning they can cause hypokalemia. Also, they can cause hypomagnesemia. Each sodium ion and chloride ion necessarily take with them a number of water molecules when they are excreted, hence the increase in urine.

Loop diuretics are sometimes called high-ceiling diuretics because they are very efficient at preventing the reabsorption of sodium, chloride, and potassium, and hence forcing the excretion of water. Loop diuretics produce more urine than other diuretics.

Furosemide can be used as monotherapy to treat hypertension or used in conjunction with other drugs. Further, furosemide treats edema resulting from heart failure, hepatic disease, and/or renal disease. Furosemide is usually dosed twice daily for most patients, but can be used twice daily when needed.

SIDE-EFFECTS

Loop diuretics can cause:
- Volume depletion
- Hypotension
- Hypokalemia
- Circulatory collapse
- Blood clots,
- Arrhythmias
- Elevate uric acid levels
- Elevate blood glucose levels
- Elevate LDL cholesterol, and
- Decrease LDL cholesterol

DRUG INTERACTIONS

NSAIDs can decrease the effectiveness of diuretics by decreasing blood flow to the kidneys. NSAIDs prevent prostaglandins from increasing renal blood flow.

THIAZIDE DIURETICS

These drugs include chlorothiazide and hydrochlorothiazide. Thiazide diuretics prevent the sodium-ion-chloride-ion symport pump from moving sodium and chloride ions from inside the distal tubules back ultimately into the blood; this causes sodium and chloride ions to be excreted, and necessarily taking water with them. Only about 10% of filtered sodium ions reach the sodium-ion-chloride-ion symport pump; therefore, thiazide diuretics can only block a limited amount of sodium ions from reabsorption; hence their limited effectiveness.

Start patients with heart failure on thiazide diuretics; switch to a more powerful loop diuretic if necessary, such as bumetanide. Thiazide diuretics are contraindicated in people with allergies to sulfonamides.

SIDE-EFFECTS

Depsitpe only 10% of sodium ions reaching the sodium-ion-chloride-ion symport pump, these drugs can cause serious depletion of sodium to the point of causing death. Long-term use of thiazide and thiazide-like diuretics may result in magnesium deficiency, especially in people at risk of poor nutrition, including some elderly. Thiazide diuretics may increase blood calcium levels.

DRUG INTERACTIONS

Thiazide diuretics and quinidine together can cause arrhythmias. Thiazide diuretics may increase levels of digoxin and lithium. In contrast, thiazide diuretics can decrease levels of warfarin and other anticoagulants, insulin, sulfonylureas, and probenecid.

POTASSIUM SPARING DIURETICS

These drugs include amiloride, eplerenone, and triamterene. Potassium-sparing diuretics work in the distal tubule. These diuretics block sodium channels (in the distal tubule) from allowing sodium to pass from inside the distal tubule to the interstitial fluid. Normally, as sodium passes from the distal tubule into the interstitial fluid, potassium flows from the interstitial fluid into the distal tubule. In this part of the nephron, sodium must pass from inside the tubule to the interstitial fluid, before potassium can pass from the interstitial fluid into the distal tubule. The blocking of these sodium channels prevents potassium from entering the distal tubule, thus "sparing" it from being urinated out of the body. The net effect is to increase urine formation.

SIDE-EFFECTS

Hyperkalemia is the most important side-effect. Avoid potassium sparing diuretics in patients with conditions that may cause hyperkalemia such as patients with renal failure.

DRUG INTERACTIONS

Avoid using potassium-sparing diuretics with drugs that cause potassium retention. These drugs include ACE inhibitors and NSAIDs. Patients on potassium sparing diuretics should avoid potassium supplements and salt alternatives that replace sodium with potassium.

NITRATES

Nitrates such as nitroglycerin, isosorbide dinitrate, and isosorbide mononitrate, release nitric oxide molecules, dilating vascular smooth muscle. This lowers the work load placed on the heart; that is they reduce the amount of oxygen that the heart needs, thus reducing the sharp pains associated with angina. Tolerance develops to nitrates, thus limiting their ability to reduce the work load placed on the heart. Prevent tolerance by instructing patients to go without nitroglycerin for at least eight hours each day.

SIDE-EFFECTS

Nitroglycerin may cause flushing of the face and headache.

DRUG INTERACTIONS

Use of nitrates with erectile dysfunction drugs sildenafil, tadalafil, or vardenafil may cause profound hypotension. Because of the profound decrease in blood pressure caused by taking these drugs together, patients should not take these drugs together.

CALCIUM CHANNEL BLOCKERS

Calcium channel blockers can be divided into two main classes: dihydropyridines (amlodipine, felodipine, and nifedipine) and non-dihydropyridines (diltiazem and verapamil). Many other calcium channel blockers exist, however these are the main ones used in clinical practice. All calcium channel blockers treat hypertension by decreasing the flow of calcium ions into vascular smooth muscle. Verapamil and diltiazem also treat paroxysmal supraventricular tachycardias and various types of angina by decreasing the flow of calcium ions into cardiac tissue. The dihydropyridines are used as antihypertensive drugs and not as antiarrhythmics.

All calcium channel blockers may cause hypotension. Hypotension may cause dizziness, leading to falls and broken bones. Because of verapamil's substantial effect on AV node conduction, it can cause bradycardia (unusually slow heart rate).

Diltiazem is contraindicated in patients with sick sinus syndrome or AV block unless the patient has a ventricular pacemaker. Diltiazem is also contraindicated in patients with hypotension or patients who have acute myocardial infarction. Using diltiazem with a beta-blocker in patients with impaired ventricular function may further decrease ventricular functioning.

Alpha Blockers - treatment of hypertension				
Generic Name	Brand Name	Dose	Mechanism of Action	Dosage Form
Doxazosin	Cardura®	Adult: 8 mg twice daily as a max dose for hypertension	Blocks alpha$_1$ receptors thus preventing adrenaline from working and raising blood pressure	Tablets 1 mg, 2 mg, 4 mg, 8 mg
Prazosin	Minipress®	Adult maintenance dose 3-15 mg two to four times daily	Dilates arteries and veins by blocking alpha$_1$ adrenergic receptors	Capsules 1 mg, 2 mg, 5 mg
Terazosin	Hytrin®	Adult maintenance dose: 1-20 mg at bedtime	Blocks alpha$_1$ receptors thus preventing adrenaline from raising blood pressure	Capsules 1 mg, 2 mg, 5 mg, 10 mg

Beta Blockers -				
Generic Name/ Brand Name	Clinical Use	Dose	Mechanism of Action	Dosage Form
Acebutolol Sectral®	Hypertension (HTN); Angina	400-1200 mg daily in two divided doses	Selectively blocks Beta$_1$ receptors	Capsules 200 mg, 400 mg
Atenolol Tenormin®	HTN, angina, heart failure	50-200 mg daily in two divided doses	Same as above	Tablets 25 mg, 50 mg, 100 mg
Betaxolol Kerlone®	HTN, angina, heart failure	10-20 mg daily	Same as above	Tablets 10 mg, 20 mg
Bisoprolol Zebeta®	HTN	2.5-5 mg daily	Same as above	Tablet 5 mg, 10 mg
Carvedilol Coreg®	HTN, angina	Adult dose 25 mg twice daily	Blocks Beta$_1$, Beta$_2$, and alpha$_1$ receptors	Tablets 2.5 mg, 6.25, 12.5 mg, 25 mg
Esmolol Brevibloc®	HTN, angina, heart failure	IV infusion 25-300 mcg/kg/min	Blocks Beta$_1$ receptors selectively	Injection 10 mg/ml
Labetalol Trandate®	HTN, angina	Adult IV continuous infusion 2 mg/minute	Blocks Beta$_1$, Beta$_2$, and alpha$_1$ receptors	Tablets 100 mg, 200 mg, 300 mg, Injection 5 mg/ml, 4 ml, 20 ml, 40 ml vials

Beta Blockers -				
Generic Name/ Brand Name	Clinical Use	Dose	Mechanism of Action	Dosage Form
Metoprolol Lopressor®	HTN, angina, heart failure	Adult 50 mg twice daily	Blocks Beta$_1$ receptors selectively	Tablets 25 mg, 50 mg, 100 mg, Extended Release tablets 25 mg, 50 mg, 100 mg
Nadolol Corgard®	HTN, angina, heart failure	Adult 40-120 mg once daily	Blocks Beta$_1$ and Beta$_2$ receptors	Tablets 20 mg, 40 mg, 80 mg, 120 mg, 160 mg
Pindolol Visken®	HTN, angina	Adult 20-60 mg once daily	Same as above	Tablets 5 mg, 10 mg
Propranolol Inderal®	HTN, angina, heart failure	Adult 80 mg twice daily	Same as above	Tabs 10 mg, 20 mg, 40 mg, 80 mg
Timolol Blocadren®	HTN, angina, heart failure, glaucoma	Adult 10 mg twice daily	Same as above	Blocadren tablets 20 mg; generic tablets 5 mg, 10 mg, 20 mg

Calcium Channel Blockers				
Non-dihydropyridines- angina, hypertension, atrial fibrillation, atrial flutter				
Generic Name	Brand Name	Dose	Mechanism of Action	Dosage Form
Diltiazem	Cardizem®, Cardizem® CD, Cardizem® LA, Cartia XT®	Adult 180-240 mg once daily	Same as above	Cardizem® CD 120 mg, 180 mg, 240 mg, 300 mg, 360 mg
Verapamil	Calan®, Calan® SR, Isoptin®, Verelan®, Verelan® PM	Adult immediate release tablets 80 mg three times daily	Inhibits calcium ions from passing through its ion channels thus relaxes cardiac smooth muscle	Tablets 80 mg, 120; Extended release tablets 120 mg, 180 mg, 240 mg

Calcium Channel Blockers - Dihydropyridines: Hypertension				
Generic Name	Brand Name	Dose	Mechanism of Action	Dosage Form
Amlodipine	Norvasc®	Adult 5-10mg once daily	Inhibits calcium ions from passing through calcium channels in cardiac cells causing a relaxation of coronary smooth muscle	Tablets 5 mg, 10 mg
Felodipine	Plendil®	Adult 2.5-10 mg once daily	Same as above	Tablets extended release 2.5 mg, 5 mg, 10 mg
Nifedipine	Procardia®, Procardia Xl®	Adult maintenance dose of 120-180 mg daily	Same as above	Procardia Xl 30 mg, 60 mg, 90 mg

Calcium Channel Blockers - Dihydropyridines: Hypertension

Generic Name	Brand Name	Dose	Mechanism of Action	Dosage Form
Isradipine	Dynacirc CR®	Adult 5-10 mg once daily	Same as above	Dynacirc® controlled release tablets 5 mg, 10 mg
Nicardipine	Cardene®	Adult capsule: 20 mg three times daily	Same as above	Cardene® capsule 20 mg, 30 mg
Nisoldipine	Sular®	Adult 10-40 mg once daily	Same as above	Tablet extended release 10 mg, 20 mg, 30 mg, 40 mg

Thiazide Diuretics - Hypertension

Generic Name	Brand Name	Dose	Mechanism of Action	Dosage Form
Chlorothiazide	Diuril®	Adult oral 250-1000 mg once to twice daily	Inhibits sodium reabsorption in the distal tubules causing increased excretion of water and potassium, meaning increased urine formation	Tablet 250 mg, 500 mg, Injection, powder for reconstitution 500 mg/vial
Hydrochlorothiazide	Microzide®	Adult oral dose 12.5-25 mg once daily	Same as above	Tablets 25 mg, Capsules 12.5 mg

Loop Diuretics - Hypertension

Generic Name	Brand Name	Dose	Mechanism of Action	Dosage Form
Bumetanide	Bumex®	Adult oral dose 0.5 mg once daily	Inhibits reabsorption of sodium and chloride in the ascending loop of Henle, causing increased urine formation	Tablets 0.5 mg, 1 mg, 2 mg
Ethacrynic Acid	Edecrin®	Adult oral dose 50-200 mg daily in divided doses	Same as above	Tablet 25 mg, Injection, powder for reconstitution 50 mg vials
Furosemide	Lasix®	Adult oral dose 20 mg once daily	Same as above	Tablets 20 mg, 40; Injection 10 mg/ml; Oral solution 10 mg/ml, 40 mg/5ml
Torsemide	Demadex®	Adult oral dose 2.5-5 mg once daily	Same as above	Tablets 5 mg, 10 mg, 20 mg, 100 mg, Injection 10 mg/ml

Potassium Sparing Diuretics - Hypertension

Generic Name	Brand Name	Dose	Mechanism of Action	Dosage Form
Amiloride	Amiloride	Adult oral dose 5-10 mg daily in one or two divided doses	Increases Na^+ excretion causing increased urine formation	Tablet 5 mg
Eplerenone	Inspra®	Adult 50 mg once to twice daily	Blocks aldosterone at its receptor in the distal tubule causing an increase in sodium and water excretion	Tablets 25 mg, 50 mg
Spironolactone	Aldactone®	Adult oral dose 25-100 mg in one or two divided doses	Same as above	Tablets 25 mg, 50 mg, 100 mg
Triamterene	Dyrenium®	Adult 100-300 mg/day in one to two divided doses	Inhibits Na^+ reabsorption, increasing in urine formation	Capsules 50 mg, 100 mg

ACE-Inhibitors Angiotensin-Converting Enzyme Inhibitor: Hypertension, heart failure, myocardial infarction, diabetic nephropathy

Generic Name	Brand Name	Dose	Mechanism of Action	Dosage Form
Benazepril	Lotensin®	Adult 5-40 mg once daily	Prevents conversion of angiotensin I to angiotensin II, angiotensin II raises blood pressure	Tablet 5 mg, 10 mg, 20 mg, 40 mg
Captopril	Capoten®	Adult 25-100mg in one to two divided doses	Same as above	Tablet 12.5 mg. 25 mg, 50 mg, 100 mg
Enalapril	Vasotec®	Adult 2.5-20 mg once daily	Same as above	Tablet 2.5 mg, 5 mg, 10 mg, 20 mg
Fosinopril	Monopril®	Adult 10-40 mg once daily	Same as above	Tablets 10 mg, 20 mg, 40 mg
Lisinopril	Prinivil®	Adult 2.5-40 mg once daily	Same as above	Tablets 2.5 mg, 5 mg, 10 mg, 20 mg, 30 mg, 40 mg
Moexipril	Univasc®	Adult 7.5-30 mg in one to two divided doses	Same as above	Tablets 7.5 mg, 15 mg
Quinapril	Accupril®	Adults 5-40 mg once daily	Same as above	Tablets 5 mg, 10 mg, 20 mg, 40 mg
Ramipril	Altace®	Adult 2.5-20 mg once daily	Same as above	Capsule 1.25 mg, 2.5 mg, 5 mg, 10 mg
Trandolapril	Mavik®	Adult 1-4 mg once daily	Same as above	Tablets 1 mg, 2 mg, 4 mg

Angiotensin Receptor II Blockers - Hypertension				
Generic Name	Brand Name	Dose	Mechanism of Action	Dosage Form
Candesartan	Atacand®	Adult 4-32 mg once daily	Blocks angiotensin II from binding with the AT1 receptor	Tablets 4 mg, 8 mg, 16 mg, 32 mg
Eprosartan	Teveten®	Adult 400-800 mg daily	Same as above	Tablet 400 mg, 600 mg
Irbesartan	Avapro®	Adult 75-300mg once daily	Same as above	Tablet 75 mg, 150 mg, 300 mg
Losartan	Cozaar®	Adult 25-100 mg once daily	Same as above	Tablet 25 mg, 50 mg, 100 mg
Olmesartan	Benicar®	Adult 5-40 mg once daily	Same as above	Tablets 5 mg, 20 mg, 40 mg
Telmisartan	Micardis®	Adult 20-80 mg once daily	Same as above	
Valsartan	Diovan®	Adult 40-320 mg once daily	Same as above	Tablets 40 mg, 80 mg, 160 mg, 320

Anti-Anginal				
Generic Name	Brand Name	Dose	Mechanism of Action	Dosage Form
Isosorbide Dinitrate	Isordil®	Adult: 5-30 mg every 8 hours	Releases nitric oxide	Generic tablets: 5 mg, 10 mg, 20 mg, and 30 mg
Isosorbide Mononitrate	Imdur®	Adult: 30-120 mg extended release tablet once in the morning	Releases nitric oxide	Tablets extended release: 30 mg, 60 mg, and 120 mg
Nitroglycerin	Nitro-dur®	Sublingual tablets: 0.4mg every 5 minutes as needed	Releases nitric oxide	Sublingual tablets 0.3 and 0.4 mg, patches, ointment, spray

Direct Vasodilators - Hypertension				
Generic Name	Brand Name	Dose	Mechanism of Action	Dosage Form
Epoprostenol	Flolan®	Adults infusion pump set at 2 ng/kg/minute	As an analog of prostacyclin, it dilates pulmonary arteries and systemic arteries, thus lowering blood pressure	Injection, powder for reconstitution 0.5 mg, 1 mg, manufacturer provides diluent
Fenoldopam	Corlopam®	Adults maximum infusion rate of 1.6 mcg/kg/minute	As a dopamine agonist at D_1 receptors, it causes renal vasodilation thus decreasing blood pressure, 6 times more potent than dopamine	Injection 10 mg/ml, 1 ml and 2 ml vials
Hydralazine	Apresoline	Adult maintenance 50 mg four times daily, max of 300 mg/day	Directly relaxes arterioles thus lowering blood pressure	Tablets 10 mg, 25 mg, 50 mg, 100 mg; Inj. 20mg/ml
Minoxidil	Loniten	Adult 2.5-80 mg in one to two divided doses	Directly relaxes arteriolar smooth muscle	Tablet 2.5 mg, 10 mg

Direct Vasodilators - Hypertension				
Generic Name	Brand Name	Dose	Mechanism of Action	Dosage Form
Nitroprusside	Nitropress®	Adults IV 3 mcg/kg/min, max 10 mcg/kg/min	Directly dilates both venous and arteriolar smooth muscle	Injection 25 mg/ml, 2 ml vials

Chapter 12

ANTI-ARRHYTHMIC DRUGS

Class I Na⁺ Channel Blockers	Class II Beta-Blockers	Class III K⁺ Channel Blockers	Class IV Ca²⁺ Channel Blockers

Class IA:
   Disopyramide
   Procainamide
   Quinidine
Class IB:
   Lidocaine
   Mexiletine
Class IC:
   Flecainide
   Moricizine
   Propafenone
	Esmolol
	Propranolol
		Amiodarone
		Dofetilide
		Ibutilide
		Sotalol
			Verapamil
			Diltiazem

Just as nerves have action potentials, cardiac cells have action potentials so the heart can beat. Action potentials are the choreographed flow of ions into and out of cardiac cells for the purpose of increasing intracellular calcium ion levels at just the right moment so the heart beats at an exact rhythm. Cardiac action potentials have five main phases. During each phase at least one ion and sometimes two ions cross the cardiac cell membrane. The five phases are: phase 0, phase 1, phase 2, phase 3, and phase 4. Phase 0 is when sodium ions rush into the cell. Phase 1 is when potassium ions rush out of the cell. Phase 2 is when calcium ions slowly enter the cell while potassium ions are still flowing out. Phase 3 involves the rapid outward flow of potassium ions. Phase 4 is when the cell is repolarized and a tiny amount of potassium ions flow out of the cell; the cell waits for pacemaker cells to re-initiate the next action potential causing a rush of sodium ions into the cell.

Arrhythmias almost always involve the heart beating too fast, but can include the heart beating too slow. Anti-arrhythmic drugs usually slow the heart rate. When the heart beats too fast, the ventricles cannot completely fill with blood, which means less blood gets pumped to the body, sometimes resulting in death.

Myocardial infarctions are probably the most common cause of arrhythmias (dead heart tissue interferes with the normal flow of electrical impulses through the heart, creating an arrhythmia).

Anti-arrhythmic drugs are divided into four main classes and a miscellaneous class. Each anti-arrhythmic class affects a different phase of cardiac action potentials. In general, by increasing the time it takes for one of the various phases of the action potential to happen, the time it takes for each beat increases, meaning less beats can occur per minute, returning the heart to it natural rate of 60 to 80 beats per minute.

Sodium channel blockers increase the time for phase 0. Beta blockers decrease the rate at which pace maker cells stimulate cardiac muscle cells, meaning the time between phase 4 and phase 0 (in part the PR interval) increases. Potassium channel blockers increase the time for phase 3 to happen. Calcium channel blockers increase the time for phase 2 and phase 4 to happen. The miscellaneous drug adenosine increases potassium flow in the AV node, thus hyperpolarizing the AV node and decreasing heart rate. Low potassium levels lead to arrhythmias. Potassium injected into the body decreases arrhythmias. Magnesium injected into the body also decreases arrhythmias.

Normal heart rhythm depends on the precise timing of the inward and outward flow of sodium ions, potassium ions, and calcium ions across cardiac cell membranes. When the natural and rhythmic flow of these ions is interrupted, an arrhythmia may occur. Arrhythmias usually result from previous injury to the heart, such as a heart attack. They can also result from genetic abnormalities. Ischemic tissue is often a source of arrhythmias. Numerous drugs exist to return the heart to its natural rhythm. Similar to antiepileptic drugs, anti-arrhythmic drugs may work by more than one mechanism, however, they are classified according to their predominant mechanism of action. Arrhythmias typically involve the heart beating faster than normal, but not always.

For conceptual purposes, anti-arrhythmic drugs are traditionally divided into five classes, Class I, Class II, Class III, Class IV, and other drugs. Class I drugs block sodium channels. Class II drugs are the already discussed beta-blockers. Class III drugs block potassium channels. Class IV drugs block calcium channels. The other drugs include adenosine, potassium, and magnesium.

Class I drugs decrease heart rate by blocking sodium channels. Sodium-channel blockers decrease the sinoatrial node's rate of firing by slowing the rate at which sodium ions pass through sodium ion channels. Slowing the rate at which sodium ions pass through sodium channels makes it take longer to reach the threshold potential at which the SA node depolarizes, thus slowing the rate of each depolarization (initiation of a new beat).

Class I drugs are traditionally divided into three subclasses based on their effects on the ventricles (the lower chambers of the heart). Class IA drugs increase the time it takes ventricle cells to repolarize. Class IB drugs shorten repolarization time. Class IC drugs do not change the total time for repolarization. Class IA drugs include procainamide, disopyramide, and quinidine. Quinidine is noted for its ability to cause torsades de pointes- a ventricular arrhythmia characterized by "twisting" of the QRS phase on an electrocardiogram (other anti-arrhythmic drugs are also capable of causing arrhythmias). Class IB drugs include lidocaine and mexiletine. Class IC drugs include flecainide, moricizine, and propafenone.

Class II anti-arrhythmic drugs are beta blockers. Esmolol, propranolol, and sotalol treat both supraventricular and ventricular arrhythmias. They block the sympathetic nervous system's signals to the sinoatrial and atrioventricular nodes. By blocking sympathetic input, beta blockers decrease the rate of depolarization, meaning less beats per minute. Second, they decrease arrhythmias by increasing the time its take to repolarize the SA node and AV node after depolarization, by making each beat take longer, the heart beats less each minute.

Class III drugs reduce arrhythmias by blocking potassium channels, increasing the time it takes for cells to repolarize, increasing each beat's duration, decreasing the amount of beats per each minute. Class III drugs include amiodarone, bretylium, ibutilide, dofetilide, and dronedarone. Ibutilide is used to end atrial fibrillation or atrial flutter. Amiodarone can treat ventricular fibrillation, and it is used to prevent paroxysmal atrial fibrillation. Amiodarone blocks both potassium channels and calcium channels, yet it also is a beta-blocker. Amiodarone does cause a wide range of side-effects including, peripheral neuropathy, headache, elevated liver enzymes, hyperthyroidism or hypothyroidism (see thyroid chapter), pulmonary fibrosis, and hypotension.

Class IV drugs are calcium channel blockers, including verapamil and diltiazem (amlodipine and nifedipine are not used for arrhythmias). They slow automaticity and conduction velocity in the AV node thus decreasing arrhythmias. They treat supraventricular arrhythmias. They can work too well, if the dose is too high, and cause AV node block. Rarely are they used to treat ventricular arrhythmias.

Adenosine treats paroxysmal supraventricular tachycardia. It does not treat atrial flutter, atrial fibrillation, or ventricular tachycardia. Adenosine decreases intracellular levels of calcium ions by inhibiting adenyl cyclase, which produces cAMP.

Anti-Arrhythmic Drugs Class 1A				
Generic Name	Brand Name	Dose	Mechanism of Action	Dosage Form
Disopyramide	Norpace®, Norpace® CR	Ventricular arrhythmias for patients greater than 50 kg: 300mg ER Q12 hours	Decreases conduction velocity through cardiac nerves, thus decreasing heart rate	Capsule 100 mg, 150 mg; Extended release capsule 100 mg, 150 mg
Procainamide	Pronestyl®	Supraventricular arrhythmias 1 gm to 1.25 gms every 6 hours	Decrease heart contractility by increasing the electrical threshold the ventricles must acquire before they can contract	Tablet 500 mg, Injection 100 mg/ml
Quinidine	Quinidine	Atrial fibrillation 300 mg to 600 mg extended release PO every 8 to 12 hours. Dosage must be individualized.	Decreases sodium influx during depolarization and decreases potassium outflow in repolarization, effectively slowing heart rate	Injection 80 mg/ml
Anti-Arrhythmic Drugs Class 1B				
Lidocaine	Xylocaine®	Adult ventricular arrhythmias: 1-4 mg/minute IV	Decreases the flow of sodium ions across the cardiac cell membrane, effectively decreases heart rate	Injection 4 mg/ml in premixed D_5W 250 ml, 500 ml bags
Mexiletine	Mexitil®	Adult 200-300 mg every 8 hours	Inhibits flow of sodium into cardiac cells, thus decreasing heart rate	Capsule 150 mg, 200 mg, 250 mg
Anti-Arrhythmic Drugs Class 1C				
Flecainide	Tambocor®	Adult ventricular arrhythmias: upto 200 mg Bid as a max dose	Slows nerve conduction in the heart by changing the transport of ions across cell membranes	Tablets 50 mg, 100 mg, 150 mg
Moricizine	Ethmozine®	Adult 200-300 mg Q8H, if needed, adjust dose after 3 days	Reduces the flow of Na^+ into the cardiac cell, thus reducing heart rate	Tablets 200 mg, 250 mg
Propafenone	Rhythmol Rhythmol SR	Adult ventricular arrhythmias: immediate release tablets 150 mg Q8H, may increase if needed	Blocks the flow of Na^+ from outside the cardiac cell to inside the cardiac cell, thus slowing the rate of increase of the action potential	Tablets 150 mg, 225 mg, 300 mg; Capsule extended release 225 mg, 325 mg, 425 mg

Anti-arrhythmic Drugs Class II Beta Blockers				
Generic Name	Brand Name	Dose	Mechanism of Action	Dosage Form
Esmolol	Brevibloc®	Adult supraventricular tachycardia: 50-200 mcg/kg/minute for next 4 minutes IV	Beta$_1$ blocker, thus decreases heart rate	Injection solution 10 mg/ml
Propranolol	Inderal®	Adult oral dose for tachyarrhythmias: 10-30 mg Q6-8H; Injection: 1-3 mg slow IV push , repeat every 2 to 5 minutes for a maximum of 5 mg.	Non-selective beta blocker, thus decreases heart rate	Tablets 10 mg, 20 mg, 40 mg, 80 mg; Injection 1mg/ml

Anti-arrhythmic Drugs Class III				
Generic Name	Brand Name	Dose	Mechanism of Action	Dosage Form
Amiodarone	Cordarone® Pacerone®	Adult maintenance dose of 400 mg QD	Inhibits adrenergic stimulation, it blocks alpha and beta receptors	Cordarone® tablets 200 mg; Pacerone® 100 mg, 200 mg, 400 mg
Dofetilide	Tikosyn®	125 mcg - 500 mcg Bid, Physicians must assess patient's QT interval first to determine whether drug can be safely used	Delays repolarization of cardiac cells thereby slowing the heart rate	Capsule 125 mcg, 250 mcg, 500 mcg
Ibutilide	Corvert®	Adults 60 kg and heavier: 1 mg over 10 minutes, if 10 minutes after end of initial dose the patient still has an arrhythmia, then may repeat once	Prolongs the action potential in cardiac cells, exactly how is unknown	Injection 0.1 mg/ml
Sotalol	Betapace®	Adult ventricular arrhythmias: initial dose 80 mg Bid; maintenance dose of 160-320 mg/day in divided doses, wait 3 days before increasing dose	Has both Class II and Class III properties. Class II properties of beta-adrenergic blocking; class III properties of prolonging cardiac action potential	Tablets 40 mg, 80 mg

Anti-arrhythmic Drugs Class IV				
Generic Name	Brand Name	Dose	Mechanism of Action	Dosage Form
Verapamil	Calan® Calan SR®	2.5-5 mg over 2 minutes; second dose of 5-10 mg may be given 15-30 minutes after first dose if needed	Slows automaticity and conduction in AV node thus decreasing arrhythmias	Injection 2.5mg/ml, 2 ml, and 4 ml vials

CHAPTER 13

ANTI-CLOTTING DRUGS

Antiplatelet Drugs	Anticoagulants			Thrombolytic Drugs
	Oral Anti-Clotting Factors	Antithrombin III Drugs	Direct Thrombin Inhibitors	
Aspirin Dipyridamole Eptifibatide Abciximab Tirofiban Clopidogrel Ticlopidine Prasugrel	Warfarin	Enoxaparin Heparin	Argatroban Bivalirudin Dabigatran Desirudin Lepirudin	Reteplase Streptokinase TPA Tenecteplase

Antiplatelet drugs and anticoagulants are used to prevent blood clots from forming. Thrombolytic drugs dissolve clots once they have formed; they are for short term use only. Platelets and coagulation factors work together to form blood clots.

Platelets depend on their surface receptors and intracellular reactions to physically stick together to form blood clots. One major receptor on the surface of platelets is the $P2Y_{12}$ receptor. Activation of this receptor is necessary for platelets to become activated so they can form clots.

Clopidogrel, ticlopidine, and prasugrel all block the $P2Y_{12}$ (adenosine diphosphate (ADP)) receptor. ADP binds at this receptor and ultimately activates platelets by decreasing protein kinase A (PKA) inside the platelet. The binding of clopidogrel, ticlopidine, or prasugrel keeps intracellular levels of PKA high, thus preventing platelets from aggregating.

Aspirin blocks the enzyme cox. Cox normally produces thromboxane A_2 (TxA_2). TxA_2 causes platelet aggregation. TxA_2 is released by activated platelets to attrack other platelets to the wound and then aggregate.

Dipyridamole, an antiplatelet drug, increases levels of cAMP within platelets, which inhibits platelet aggregation. Dipyridamole inhibits the enzyme phosphodiesterase, preventing the metabolism of cAMP, thus keeping cAMP levels high, and, consequently PKA levels high, which inhibits platelet clotting. Hepat-

ic failure has occured with the use of dipyridamole. Administration of dipyridamole with warfarin has not caused bleeding problems, but does not mean that it cannot theoretically happen.

Warfarin blocks the liver from producing clotting factors which are necessary for the production of fibrin. Fibrin is a protein. It forms long fibrous chains and mixes with aggregated platelets to complete the formation of a blood clot. Warfarin blocks the enzyme vitamin K epoxide reductase from producing the reduced form of vitamin K. The reduced form of vitamin K is necessary to produce clotting factors II, VII, IX, and X. Without these clotting factors, proper clot formation cannot occur.

Warfarin is highly bound to plasma proteins. Other drugs highly binding with plasma proteins may displace warfarin from albumin. Since warfarin is about 97-99% bound to albumin, even the slightest displacement of warfarin may double its plasma concentration. Other drugs highly bound to albumin include, methotrexate, NSAIDS, levothyroxine, and sulfonylureas.

Warfarin does not begin to work for about 24 hours. Because of this, warfarin is generally administered together with heparin or enoxaparin until a stable INR can be achieved. The INR is a measure of how long it takes for a patient's blood to clot. An INR of 2 to 3 is the range for most clinical conditions. Foods containing high amounts of vitamin K can interfere with warfarin. Patients do not need to avoid foods high in vitamin K, but they need to eat a consistent diet of foods containing vitamin K. An inconsistent diet makes it difficult to find a dose that keeps the patient's INR within the necessary range (2 to 3 for most patients).

Abciximab, eptifibatide, and tirofiban work by blocking the GPIIb/IIIa receptor on platelets. This receptor normally binds with fibrinogen. Fibrinogen is a large molecule that has multiple binding sites. Because of its multiple binding sites, fibrinogen is capable of binding with multiple platelets - this forms a large clump of platelets occluding the wound.

Abciximab, eptifibatide, and tirofiban are all contraindicated in patients with a recent history of bleeding diathesis. Further they are contraindicated in patients with severe hypertension. Hypertension puts patients at risk of stroke. All are administered intravenously.

Heparin is normally made by the body to limit clotting. Once thrombin has served its purpose of converting fibrinogen to fibrin and a clot has formed, the body needs to stop thrombin from working. Heparin works by increasing the efficiency of antithrombin III, the enzyme which is responsible for stopping thrombin from converting fibrinogen to fibrin. Heparin is administered as an IV or subcutaneous injection.

Heparin causes thrombocytopenia. Further, heparin may cause thrombosis in some patients. These patients should use the newer lower molecular weight heparins: enoxaparin and fondaparinux.

Enoxaparin and fondaparinux have the same mechanism of action as heparin and have a lower incidence of thrombocytopenia and thrombosis. Heparin, enoxaparin, and fondaparinux are administered by injection.

Direct thrombin inhibitors include argatroban, bivalirudin, dabigatran, lepirudin, and desirudin. They work by binding directly with thrombin's active site, preventing thrombin from performing its functions, such as converting fibrinogen to fibrin; activating factor XIII (factor XIII joins fibrin molecules together to form long chains); and activating platelets.

Bivalirudin inhibits thrombin by binding with the catalytic site and the anion-binding exosite of thrombin, regardless of whether thrombin is circulating or bound to clots. It is approved for patients with unstable angina undergoing percutaneous transluminal coronary angioplasty (PTCA), and for patients undergoing percutaneous coronary intervention (PCI). Bleeding is a common adverse reaction. However, it may cause less bleeding than heparin. It is contraindicated in patients with active bleeding.

Argatroban is indicated to prevent or treat clots in patients who have heparin-induced thrombocytopenia (HIT). It is also approved for PCI in patients with HIT or at risk of HIT. It is contraindicated in patients with major bleeding. It is administered as continuous IV infusion. Common adverse reactions include dyspnea, hypotension, fever, diarrhea, sepsis, and cardiac arrest.

Dabigatran is approved to lower the risk of stroke and systemic embolism for patients with non-valvular atrial fibrillation. Its dose is decreased for patients with reduced creatine clearance. More than 15% of patients experience bleeding as a side-effect. It is contraindicated in patients with active bleeding or who have a mechanical prosthetic heart valve.

Thrombolytic drugs dissolve clots that have already formed. The above drugs are not effective at dissolving already formed clots. Streptokinase, tissue plasminogen activator (TPA), reteplase, and tenecteplase all dissolve clots. They work by binding with plasminogen and converting it to plasmin. Plasmin dissolves blood clots.

TPA binds with plasminogen but only if part of it is also bound to fibrin; this limits TPA to working at the location of a clot. TPA is naturally produced in the body. Tenecteplase is a version of TPA produced by recombinant DNA technology. By altering the molecule, its half-life is increased. Its initial half-life is 20 to 24 minutes. Its terminal half-life is 90 to 130 minutes. It is approved to treat acute myocardial infarction. It is contraindicated in patients with active bleeding, history of cerebrovascular accident, intracranial or intraspinal surgery or trauma within 2 months, intracranial neoplasm, arteriovenous malformation, or aneurysm, known bleeding diathesis, or severe uncontrolled hypertension (package insert). Streptokinase may cause anaphylaxis, and, consequently is not used that much anymore.

Anti-Clotting Drugs				
Generic Brand	Clinical Use	Contraindications	Adverse Effects	Dosing
Aspirin	Reduce risk of myocardial infarction, transient ischemic attack, or thromboembolic disorders; acute coronary syndrome (ACS)	Bronchospasm caused by aspirin allergy; hypersensitivity to salicylates; bleeding disorders; pregnancy	Ulcers, bleeding, hemorrhage	81 mg to 325 mg daily
Dipyridamole / Aspirin Aggrenox®	Reduce risk of stroke for patients who have a history of transient ischemia of brain or thrombosis that caused ischemic stroke	Hypersensitivity to dipyridamole or ingredients	Headache and dizziness	Dipyridamole 200 mg and Aspirin 25 mg in one capsule administered twice daily
Thienopyridines				
Clopidogrel Plavix®	Prevent clots in patients with recent myocardial infarction, stroke, or established peripheral vascular disease; ACS	Bleeding (ulcers)	Rash Bleeding Bruising	75 mg orally once daily
Prasugrel Effient®	Reduce risk of cardiovascular events (includes stent thrombosis) for patients with ACS who will undergo PCI	Bleeding	Atrial fibrillation, bleeding, bradycardia, hypertension, leukopenia	Loading dose of 60 mg then 10 mg orally once daily. 75 mg to 325 mg of aspirin should also be given
Ticlopidine (Not a drug of choice, clopidogrel is favored)	Reduce risk of thrombotic stroke, reduce risk of stent thrombosis	Bleeding (ulcers) Intracranial hemorrhage; hepatic dysfunction, neutropenia	Diarrhea	250 mg orally twice daily
Glycoprotein IIb/IIIa Receptor Antagonists				
Abciximab Reopro®	Adjunct treatment for percutaneous coronary intervention (PCI) to prevent cardiac ischemic complications	Bleeding diathesis coadministration with eptifibatide or tirofiban	Acute thrombocytopenia	IV bolus of 0.25 mg/kg bolus given 10 to 60 minutes before PCI then 0.125 mcg/kg/minute for 12 hours (max of 10 mcg/minute)

Anti-Clotting Drugs				
Generic Brand	Clinical Use	Contraindications	Adverse Effects	Dosing
Eptifibatide Integrilin®	ACS; PCI	Abnormal bleeding within 30 days History of bleeding diathesis Uncontrolled hypertension	Bleeding Hypotension	ACS 180 mcg/kg (maximum of 22.6 mg) over 1 to 2 minutes, then continuous infusion of 2 mcg/kg/min (max 15 mg hour until discharge or CABG
Tirofiban Aggrastat®	Treats ACS with heparin	Bleeding History of bleeding diathesis within 30 days; stroke; recent major surgery	Active internal bleeding; severe hypertension; history of bleeding diathesis within 30 days; major surgery within prior month	IV 0.4 mcg/kg/minute for 30 minutes, then 0.1 mcg/kg/minute, continue for 12 to 24 hours after angioplasty
Vitamin K Epoxide Reductase Antagonist				
Warfarin Coumadin®	Prophylaxis and treatment venous thrombosis, pulmonary emboli; prevent and treat thromboembolic complications from atrial fibrillation and/or cardiac valve replacement; reduce risk of death, recurrent myocardial infarction (MI) or clotting after initial MI	Pregnancy Hemorrhagic tendencies or blood dyscrasias; Major surgery including eye surgery; bleeding tendencies; spinal puncture; malignant hypertension	Hemorrhage	Doses vary considerably from 0.5 mg daily to 20 mg daily. Most doses between 1 mg and 10 mg
Antithrombin III Drugs				
Heparin	Pulmonary embolism; deep vein thrombosis; unstable angina	Bleeding History of heparin induced thrombocytopenia; hematoma	Bleeding Hemorrhage Bruising Thrombocytopenia	IV infusion loading dose of 80 units/kg then continuous IV infusion of 18 units/kg/hour (ACCP)

Anti-Clotting Drugs

Generic Brand	Clinical Use	Contraindications	Adverse Effects	Dosing
Enoxaparin Lovenox®	Prophylaxis deep vein thrombosis for various surgeries; inpatient treatment of acute DVT without PE; acute ST elevated myocardial infarction; unstable angina or non Q wave myocardial infarction	Active major bleeding; thrombocytopenia linked with a positive in vitro test for anti-platelet antibody	Hemorrhage Thrombocytopenia Fever Pain	ST- elevation myocardial infarction 30 mg IV bolus plus 1 mg/kg Subcutaneous, then 1 mg/kg subcutaneous every 12 hours for patients under 75. For patients over 75 0.75 mg/kg every 12 hours (manufacturer recommends max of 75 mg for 1st two doses for patients 75 and older)

Direct Thrombin Inhibitors

Generic Brand	Clinical Use	Contraindications	Adverse Effects	Dosing
Argatroban	Prophylaxis or treatment of thrombosis in patients with heparin induced thrombocytopenia	Active major bleeding. Use with caution in patients with severe liver dysfunction	Chest pain Hypotension	Obtain baseline aPTT. Heparin induced thrombocytopenia: 2 mcg/kg/minute (max of 10 mcg/kg/minute). Adjust dose until aPTT is 1.5 to 3 times initial baseline
Bivalirudin Angiomax®	Patients with unstable angina undergoing percutaneous transluminal coronary angioplasty (PTCA), (PCI)	Active major bleeding;	Bleeding Hemorrhage Thrombocytopenia	PTCA or PCI 0.75 mg/kg bolus right before procedure then 1.75 mg/kg/hour during procedure and for 4 hours more if needed
Dabigatran Pradaxa®	Stroke and reduce risk of embolism	Bleeding Mechanical prosthetic heart valve	Bleeding	150 mg orally twice daily. Doses must be adjusted for decreased kidney functioning

CHAPTER 14

ANTI-LIPID DRUGS

Bile Acid Sequestrants	HMG-CoA Reductase Inhibitors (Statins)	Fibric Acid Derivatives	Inhibitors of Cholesterol Absorption
Colesevelam Colestipol Cholestyramine	Atorvastatin Lovastatin Pravastatin Rosuvastatin Simvastatin	Fenofibrate Gemfibrozil	Ezetimib

Cholesterol and triglycerides both affect the cardiovascular system. They may harden and thicken artery walls. They may contribute to heart attacks and strokes. LDL cholesterol levels above 130 require treatment. Various factors determine when therapy for high triglycerides should be started. Statins decrease the production of cholesterol by inhibiting HMG-CoA reductase, one of the enzymes involved in cholesterol production. Ezetimib inhibits intestinal cells from absorbing dietary cholesterol. Bile acid sequestrants sequester bile acid in the intestinal tract, thus preventing them from circulating back into the liver; normally bile acids circulate between the GI tract and liver so they can be used over and over. By interrupting this endless cycling, bile acid sequestrants force the liver to use cholesterol to produce more bile acids. Bile acids are used to aid in digestion and eliminate waste products in feces. Niacin prevents the production of fatty acids, which in turn prevents the production of triglycerides. Fibric acid derivatives increase the metabolism of fatty acids, thus preventing them from being used to produce triglycerides. Many patients require the administration of at least two drugs from the above classes to adequately control cholesterol and triglyceride levels.

The statins may cause myopathy, a type of muscle pain. Usually this can be reversed by stopping the drug. However, in some cases the pain does not end even when drug therapy ends.

The word "lipid" (fat) includes: single chain fatty acid molecules, triglycerides (which are three fatty acid molecules joined together by glycerol), and, finally, cholesterol. Cholesterol is not chemically or technically a fat or lipid, but the body makes cholesterol from triglycerides (which are fats), consequently, it is often labeled a "fat." Excess lipids and cholesterol cause atherosclerosis. This is the formation of fatty plaques on the inside of blood vessels. These fatty plaques can cause heart attacks and may contribute to causing blood clots.

Lipids and cholesterol do not float around in the blood all alone because they are too hydrophobic to dissolve in blood, which is mostly aqueous (water) based. Rather, they are transported from the intestinal tract and the liver to muscles and fat cells by molecules called "lipoproteins." Lipoproteins come in a variety of sizes. From largest to smallest in size, they are chylomicrons (CM), very-low-density lipoprotein (VLDL), intermediate-density lipoprotein (IDL), low-density lipoprotein (LDL), and high-density lipoprotein (HDL). CM form in the intestines and transport triglycerides that are eaten. The liver produces VLDL which transports triglycerides to muscles to be used as a source of energy (ATP production) or transports triglycerides to fat cells where it will be stored as fat, waiting to be used as energy. VLDL is converted to IDL which in turn is converted into LDL or HDL. Each conversion results in a progressively smaller lipoprotein.

The goals of drug therapy are to decrease the amount triglycerides and cholesterol in the bloodstream. Anti-lipid drugs include bile acid sequestrants, fibric acid derivatives, nicotinic acid, HMG-CoA reductase inhibitors (also called "statins"), and inhibitors of cholesterol absorption. By various mechanisms of action, these drugs ultimately lower blood levels of LDL-C ("bad cholesterol," low-density-lipoprotein cholesterol).

BILE ACID SEQUESTRANTS

Colesevelam, colestipol, and cholestyramine are indicated to reduce elevated LDL cholesterol in patients with primary hypercholesterolemia (Fredrickson Type

IIa). Bile acid sequestrants bind with bile acids, causing them to be removed in the stool, as opposed to being reabsorbed back into the liver. The liver must now use cholesterol from the blood and liver to produce new bile acids, thus the amount of cholesterol in the body declines. Because the liver needs cholesterol from the blood to produce more bile acids, it increases the amount of receptors that bind LDL-C, thus increasing the amount of LDL-C withdrawn from the blood.

SIDE-EFFECTS

The most common side-effects are constipation, flatulence, and dyspepsia.

DRUG INTERACTIONS

These drugs prevent the absorption of many other drugs. Patients should separate cholestyramine from other drugs by at least 2 hours, if not 4 hours. Bile acid sequestrants strongly bind niacin; consequently niacin should be given 4 to 6 hours after administration of bile acid sequestrants.

NIACIN

Niacin inhibits the production of triglycerides by inhibiting the synthesis of fatty acids (three fatty acid molecules make up a triglyceride molecule).

SIDE-EFFECTS

Niacin can cause intense facial flushing. Some patients can reduce these symptoms by taking an aspirin about 30 minutes before; some people can reduce flushing by taking niacin with a snack. Other people require a long-acting form of niacin. Others may discontinue niacin because of the flushing.

DRUG INTERACTIONS

Niacin and statins when given together increase the risk of myopathy and rhabdomyolysis.

HMG-COA REDUCTASE INHIBITORS

HMG-CoA reductase inhibitors prevent the enzyme HMG-CoA reductase from turning HMG-CoA into mevalonic acid, a precursor in the synthesis of cholesterol. Atorvastatin, lovastatin, pravastatin, rosuvastatin, and simvastatin are commonly used statins.

SIDE-EFFECTS

HMG-CoA reductase inhibitors can elevate liver enzyme levels, particularly alanine aminotransferase (ALT). Further, statins may cause myopathy and rhabdomyolysis, a more severe form of myopathy. Myopathy is defined as muscle pain or weakness together with a creatine kinase (CK) level ten times the normal upper limit. Rhabdomyolysis, a more severe form of myopathy, characterized by muscle breakdown causing myoglobinuria, may cause renal failure and death.

DRUG INTERACTIONS

Inhibitors of CYP3A4, erythromycin, fluconazole, cyclosporine, and amiodarone, all may increase levels of statins; however pravastatin is not substantially metabolized by this enzyme. Additionally, niacin and statins when given together increase the risk of myopathy and rhabdomyolysis.

FIBRIC ACID DERIVATIVES

Fibric acid derivatives, such as gemfibrozil and fenofibrate, bind as agonists with the peroxisome proliferator-activated receptors (PPARs). Activation of PPAR may in turn increase production of lipoprotein lipase, increasing metabolism of triglycerides. (Single chain fatty-acids can either be metabolized to produce energy or, second, turned into triglycerides, a form of stored energy, excess triglycerides are harmful). Gemfibrozil is for adult patients with very high elevations of serum triglycerides (Types IV and V hyperlipidemia; > 2000 mg/dL). Fenofibrate is indicated to reduce hypercholesterolemia and hypertriglyceridemia. Fenofibrate and gemfibrozil are contraindicated in patients with hepatic or severe renal dysfunction or preexisting gallbladder disease.

SIDE-EFFECTS

About one-third of patients experience gastrointestinal side-effects with gemfibrozil. Increases in abnormal liver function tests is the most common side-effects associated with fenofibrate.

DRUG INTERACTIONS

Do not administer gemfibrozil with repaglinide. Gemfibrozil and HMG-Co-A reductase inhibitors are both metabolized by the same enzyme (glucuronosyl transferases); the concurrent administration of both drugs may be too much for this enzyme to handle, thus resulting in greater blood concentrations of both drugs, and thus leading to myopathy. Gemfibrozil also reduces the transport of some statins (the organic acids) into the liver, thus also leading to elevated blood levels of statins. Fenofibrate also may cause myopathy.

Further, gemfibrozil and fenofibrate may interfere with anticoagulant medications; close monitoring is advised until the prothrombin time has definitively stabilized.

INHIBITORS OF CHOLESTEROL ABSORPTION

Ezetimib inhibits the small intestine from absorbing cholesterol by 54%. It blocks the sterol transporter: Niemann-Pick C1-Like 1. This causes the liver to use its own storage of cholesterol and to also remove cholesterol from the blood. Ezetimibe is often used in conjunction with other cholesterol lowering drugs, including simvastatin. Ezetimibe is not recommended for patients who have moderate or severe hepatic impairment.

SIDE EFFECTS

Ezetimibe rarely raises hepatic transaminase levels. Ezetimibe is well tolerated overall.

DRUG INTERACTIONS

Ezetimibe and cyclosporine increase each other's blood levels. Cyclosporine levels should be monitored in patients receiving ezetimibe. Cholestyramine substantially decreases ezetimibe levels. Ezetimibe may alter the affects of warfarin; consequently the International Normalized Ratio (INR) should be monitored closely.

HMG-CoA Reductase Inhibitors: Reduce Cholesterol Synthesis				
Generic Name	Brand Name	Dose	Mechanism of Action	Dosage Form
Atorvastatin	Lipitor®	10-80 mg QHS	Blocks HMG-CoA Reductase decreasing cholesterol synthesis and decreasing VLDL	Tablets 10 mg, 20 mg, 40 mg, 80 mg
Lovastatin	Mevacor®	10-40 mg QHS	Same as above	Tablets 10 mg, 20 mg, 40, also available as extended release
Pravastatin	Pravachol®	10-80 mg QHS	Same as above	Tablets 10 mg, 20 mg, 40 mg, 80 mg
Rosuvastatin	Crestor®	5-40 mg QHS	Same as above	Tablets 5 mg, 10 mg, 20 mg, 40 mg
Simvastatin	Zocor®	5-80 mg QHS	Same as above	Tablets 5 mg, 10 mg, 20 mg, 40 mg, 80 mg.

Anti-Triglycerides and/or Cholesterol Lowering Drugs				
Generic Name	Brand Name	Dose	Mechanism of Action	Dosage Form
Cholestyramine	Questran®	4 gms QD-Bid, max of 24 gms/24hours	Binds bile acids causing the body to increase LDL receptors and convert cholesterol to bile acid as a compensatory mechanism	Questran®: 4 gms of resin in 9 gm packet; Questran® can with 378 gms
Colesevelam	Welchol®	3 Tablets Bid with meals or 6 tablets QD with a meal	Bind bile acids causing their excretion and consequently increase LDL receptors in the liver	Tablet 625mg
Colestipol	Colestid®	Tablets initial dose of 2 gms QD-BID, increase by 2 gms at 1-2 month intervals	Same as above	Tablet 1 gm; Granules in packets of 5 gm active ingredient
Fenofibrate	Antara® Lofibra® Tricor®	Tricor 48 - 145 mg QD	Activates peroxisome proliferator-activated receptor increasing lipoprotein lipase activity, increasing metabolism of triglycerides	Tricor® tablets 48 mg, 145 mg; Lofibra® capsules 67 mg, 134 mg, 200 mg
Gemfibrozil	Lopid®	1 tablet Bid, 30 minutes before breakfast and dinner	Same as above	Tablet 600 mg
Omega-3-Acid Ethyl Esters	Lovaza®	2 capsules Bid	Increase metabolism of cholesterol	Capsule 1 gm
Niacin	Niaspan®	500-2000 mg QHS as tolerated, titrate by 500 mg every 4 weeks	Lowers triglyceride levels and may increase LDL-C	Niaspan® 500 mg, 750 mg, 1000mg

CHAPTER 15

NSAIDS, ANTI-RHEUMATOID, ARTHRITIS DRUGS, AND ANTI-GOUT DRUGS

Non-Steroidal Anti-Inflammatory Drugs		Disease Modifying Anti-Rheumatic Drugs (DMARDs)		Anti-Gout
Ibuprofen	Flurbiprofen	Small Molecules:	Biologicals:	Colchicine
Meloxicam	Indomethacin	Azathioprine	Abatacept	Allopurinol
Naproxen	Ketorolac	Cyclophosphamide	Adalimumab	Febuxostat
Diclofenac	Nabumetone	Cyclosporine	Anakinra	Probenecid
Diflunisal	Piroxicam	Hydroxychloroquine	Certolizumab	
Etodolac	Sulindac	Leflunomide	Golimumab	
	Celecoxib	Methotrexate	Infliximab	
		Sulfasalazine	Rituximab	

Non-steroidal anti-inflammatory drugs (NSAIDs) treat inflammation associated with a wide variety of causes, including arthritis, gout, and physical injuries. NSAIDs work by blocking the enzymes cox-1 and cox-2 from producing prostaglandins. Cox-1 produces beneficial prostaglandins that protect the body, including protecting the stomach. Cox-2 produces prostaglandins that cause fever and pain and inflammation. Older NSAIDs block both cox-1 and cox-2. Celecoxib, a newer NSAID, blocks cox-2. Celecoxib produces less stomach side-effects for some patients. NSAIDs are used to treat arthritis, but they are not effective at preventing joint damage.

Disease modifying anti-rheumatic drugs (DMARDs) decrease the immune system's attack on joints. DMARDs are effective at decreasing joint damage (that is the basis for calling them "disease modifying").

Rheumatoid arthritis is an auto-immune disease. Hence the basis for all DMARDs is that they decrease the immunes system's attack on joints. Small molecules, which are small organic drugs, decrease the overall activity of immune cells. Methotrexate, azathioprine, and leflunomide all interfere with the production of DNA, thus decreasing the production of some immune cells, thus decreasing the immune system's ability to attack joints. Some biologicals work by blocking tumor necrosis factor alpha (TNF-alpha). TNF-alpha causes macrophages to destroy joint tissue.

As expected, because they decrease the functioning of the immune system, DMARDs leave the body susceptible to infection. Methotrexate must not be administered every day because it will be fatal.

Anti-gout drugs work by decreasing the production of uric acid; increasing the urinary excretion of uric acid; and decreasing the immune system's attack on uric acid, which is responsible for the pain and inflammation associated with gout.

NON-STEROIDAL ANTI-INFLAMMATORY DRUGS

NSAIDs inhibit the enzymes cyclooxygenase-1 (cox-1) and cyclooxygenase-2 (cox-2), which are responsible for producing prostaglandins. Prostaglandins produced by cox-2 cause inflammation, pain, and fever. Prostaglandins produced by cox-1 protect the stomach lining. Older NSAIDs inhibit both cox-1 and cox-2; thus causing severe GI problems in some patients (although meloxicam is relatively selective for cox-2). Celecoxib is selective for cox-2. NSAIDS work in all areas of the body.

Commonly used NSAIDs include ibuprofen, meloxicam, naproxen, and diclofenac. NSAIDs treat pain, inflammation, and fever. NSAIDs are commonly used to treat osteoarthritis and rheumatoid arthritis. Ketorolac is used for 3 to 5 days after surgery because of its strong analgesic characteristics. Ketorolac can cause fatal gastrointestinal bleeding, and is therefore limited to 5 days of use.

NSAIDS are traditionally divided into 5 classes based on their chemical structure: 1) proprionic acid, 2) acetic acid, 3) ketone, 4) oxicam, and 5) fenamate analogs (aspirin is considered to occupy its own class). The generic name of a NSAID tells you which class it is in. For example, ibuprofen is in the proprionic acid class; the "pro" in ibuprofen indicates proprionic acid; all proprionic acid derivatives have "pro" in the name. Further, acetic acid derivatives have "ac" in the name: diclofenac, etodolac, indomethacin, ketorolac, and sulindac. Although, two NSAIDs may in different classes based on chemical structure that does not mean that they cannot treat the same condition. For example, ibuprofen and diclofenac can both be used to treat arthritis.

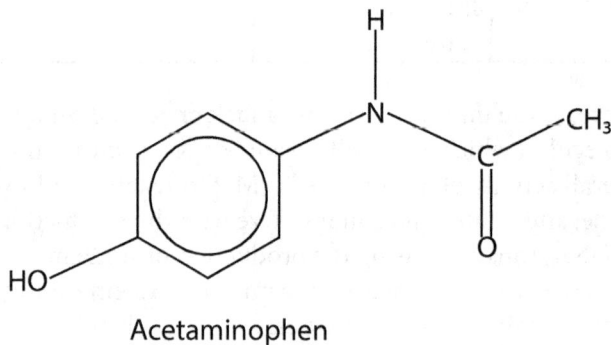

Acetaminophen

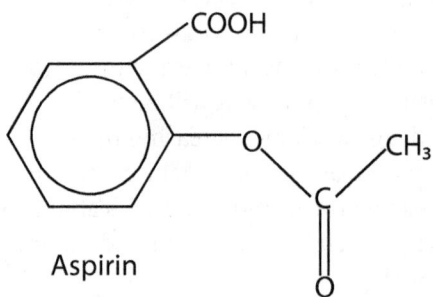

Aspirin

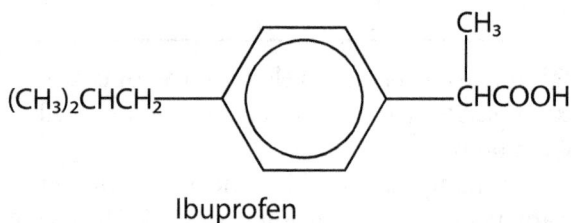

Ibuprofen

ADVERSE EFFECTS

NSAIDS cause a variety of adverse effects. NSAIDs can adversely affect the gastrointestinal tract, kidneys, heart, central nervous system, uterus, and platelets. Prostaglandins protect the stomach from stomach acid. A decrease in the production of prostaglandins in the stomach may lead to ulcers. COX-1 is responsible for producing prostaglandins in the stomach, consequently, NSAIDs that are selective for COX-2 may cause less gastrointestinal side-effects. Misoprostol, a prostaglandin E-1 replacement, reduces the damage caused by NSAIDS to the GI tract. Furthermore, proton-pump inhibitors also may prevent ulcers in some patients receiving a NSAID. Occasionally, anemia results from gastrointestinal bleeding. Additional GI side-effects include nausea, abdominal pain, and diarrhea.

Long-term use of high doses of NSAIDs can cause kidney failure; however, this is reversible if use is stopped early enough. NSAIDs reduce renal blood flow by reducing the production of prostaglandins influencing renal blood flow.

Also, NSAIDs have the ability to increase the risk of heart attack and stroke. Heart attack or stroke may result from clotting. Prostacyclin, one of the participants inhibiting clotting, depends on COX-2 for its production. NSAIDs, as COX-2 inhibitors, detrimentally block the production of prostacyclin. Consequently, NSAIDs may increase the risk of clot formation, leading to a heart attack or stroke.

DRUG INTERACTIONS

NSAIDs interact with several different drugs in clinically important ways. NSAIDs and aspirin together may increase the risk of gastrointestinal bleeding. NSAIDs, displace warfarin, methotrexate, and sulfonylurea drugs from plasma albumin, thus increasing the amount of active drug, thus increasing adverse effects. This displaced drug is the functional equivalent of giving the patient an overdose. The co-administration of an NSAID with methotrexate has resulted in fatalities.

Indomethacin, ibuprofen, naproxen, and piroxicam may increase plasma concentrations of lithium, an agent used for bipolar disorders, by inhibiting its renal excretion and promoting its reabsorption. Conversely, sulindac, another NSAID, may decrease or increase lithium plasma levels. Lithium, a narrow therapeutic index drug, is generally effective and safe between serum concentrations of 0.6-1.5 mEq/L.

ANTI-RHEUMATOID ARTHRITIS DRUGS

Rheumatoid arthritis, an autoimmune disease, persistently inflames joints, ruining and deforming them. Treatment entails decreasing inflammation, thus preventing joint deformation. NSAIDs decrease inflammation in most patients, however, NSAIDs are not strong enough to prevent joint deformation. Disease-modifying anti-rheumatic drugs (DMARDs) are designed to prevent and limit joint deformation by decreasing inflammation. DMARDs are subdivided into two classes: biologicals and non-biologicals, sometimes referred to as "small molecules. Small molecules include drugs such as azathioprine, cyclophosphamide, cyclosporine, hydroxychloroquine, leflunomide, methotrexate, minocycline, and sulfasalazine. Biologicals include abatacept, adalimumab, anakinra, certolizumab, golimumab, infliximab, and rituximab.

SMALL MOLECULES

METHOTREXATE

Methotrexate hinders the progression of arthritis, exactly how this occurs is unknown, but it probably reduces the number of immune cells attacking joints and deforming them. Methotrexate reduces the synthesis of folic acid. Folic acid provides necessary building blocks (hydroxymethyl groups and formyl groups) for the synthesis of DNA; without these building blocks, the body produces less immune cells to attack joints. Methotrexate is a last choice because of its severe side-effects.

ADVERSE REACTIONS

Methotrexate reduces bone marrow production of blood cells. This can be fatal. Calcium leucovorin is an antidote for methotrexate. It is used to treat hematological crisis caused by methotrexate suppressing bone marrow functioning. Because of the possibility of hematological crisis, a patient's CBC should be taken before initiation of methotrexate treatment and periodically thereafter.

Methotrexate has a black box warning about it potentially causing hepatic damage. A baseline liver biopsy should be taken for patients who have risk factors for developing hepatic fibrosis. These risk factors include alcohol abuse, hepatitis B, and/or hepatitis C. Methotrexate should be avoided in patients who already have hepatic fibrosis, substantially abnormal liver function tests, or other liver diseases. A liver biopsy should be taken in patients who have reached a total cumulative dose of 1-1.5 grams.

DRUG INTERACTIONS

Methotrexate is highly bound to albumin, and consequently displaces other drugs that are highly bound to plasma proteins, including warfarin, sulfonamides, salicylates, and phenytoin. NSAIDs inhibit the renal excretion of methotrexate; this can lead to the fatal accumulation of methotrexate. Proton pump inhibitors may increase methotrexate blood levels when methotrexate is administered at high doses.

AZATHIOPRINE

By suppressing lymphocytes, azathioprine diminishes the damage caused by lymphocytes, a type of white blood cell. Azathioprine, an antimetabolite for purines, inhibits the synthesis of purines. Purines are needed to synthesize DNA. Without DNA synthesis, cells, such as lymphocytes, cannot function. Azathioprine is also used to prevent rejection of transplanted organs.

ADVERSE EFFECTS

Azathioprine suppresses bone marrow production of white blood cells (leukopenia). It also suppresses production of platelets (thrombocytopenia). It has the potential to cause anemia. As it suppresses the immune system, azathioprine makes the body more vulnerable to infections.

DRUG INTERACTIONS

The liver metabolizes azathioprine to several active metabolites. These active metabolites are in turn metabolized by an enzyme called xanthine oxidase. Xanthine oxidase metabolizes the active metabolites of azathioprine into inactive metabolites. Allopurinol, an antigout drug, inhibits xanthine oxidase from working. This causes the buildup of azathioprine-active metabolites when azathioprine and allopurinol are administered together. Co-administration of allopurinol necessitates a 75% reduction in the dose of azathioprine.

CYCLOSPORINE

Cyclosporine suppresses T-lymphocytes. T-lymphocytes play a role in the pathogenesis of rheumatoid arthritis. By suppressing T-lymphocytes, cyclosporine reduces the progression of arthritic damage. Specifically, cyclosporine prevents antigens from causing T-lymphocytes to produce lymphokines. Lymphokines normally stimulate the rest of the immune system, but this does not happen with cyclosporin.

ADVERSE EFFECTS

Although very little cyclosporine is eliminated through the kidneys, cyclosporine prevents the kidneys from functioning properly and causes nephrotoxicity, which frequently leads to discontinuance of cyclosporine treatment. Further, cyclosporine frequently causes hypertension in patients who have had kidney or heart transplants.

DRUG INTERACTIONS

CYP3A isoenzymes extensively metabolize cyclosporine. Drugs inhibiting CYP3A increase blood levels of cyclosporine. These drugs include fluconazole, ketoconazole, erythromycin, indinavir, and allopurinol. Drugs inducing CYP3A decrease blood concentrations of cyclosporine. These drugs include rifampin, phenytoin, phenobarbital, carbamazepine, griseofulvin, and fosphenytoin. Grapefruit juice, an inhibitor of CYP3A, may increase blood levels of cyclosporine.

LEFLUNOMIDE

Leflunomide inhibits the synthesis of pyrimidines, which prevents the normal functioning of T-lymphocytes. T-lymphocytes produce interleukin-2, which activates other areas of the immune system. Without interleukin-2, the immune system remains suppressed and less damage to joints occurs.

ADVERSE EFFECTS

Leflunomide commonly causes respiratory tract infections and diarrhea. It may cause hypertension in about ten percent of patients. Although not common, leflunomide has caused hepatic failure and death. Therefore, leflunomide should be cautiously used in patients with liver disease. Because of liver toxicity, leflunomide should be used cautiously, if at all, with other drugs that are hepatotoxic. Further, because of fetal risks, leflunomide is contraindicated in female patients who are not reliably using birth control.

BIOLOGICALS

As a group, biologicals that treat rheumatoid arthritis work by decreasing various elements of the immune system. Tumor necrosis factor blockers bind with tumor necrosis factor-alpha (TNF-alpha), preventing TNF from binding with TNF receptors. TNF-alpha causes macrophages to destroy joint tissue. Consequently, tumor necrosis factor blockers limit the damage done to joints. These drugs include adalimumab, certolizumab, etanercept, infliximab, and golimumab. These drugs all bind with TNF preventing it from binding with its receptor.

All drugs blocking TNF-alpha make the body susceptible to infections because they depress the immune system. Respiratory infections commonly occur in patients treated with inhibitors of TNF-alpha. Further, TNF-alpha inhibitors can reactivate dormant tuberculosis, and allow new tuberculosis infections. Similarly, because TNF-alpha kills tumor cells, inhibitors of TNF-alpha may increase the risk of developing tumors. Inhibitors of TNF-alpha also can aggravate congestive heart failure.

T cells are responsible for considerable damage in rheumatoid arthritis. T cells have a receptor on their cell surface called CD28. Activation of T cells requires CD28 to bind with the ligands CD80 and CD86 on antigen presenting cells. Abatacept binds with CD80 and CD86, thus preventing antigen presenting cells from activating T cells. This has the added benefit of decreasing production of TNF-alpha. Other anti-rheumatoid drugs, such as, methotrexate, NSAIDs, corticosteroids, or drugs blocking TNF-alpha, do not affect elimination of abatacept.

Anakinra competitively inhibits interleukin-1 (IL-1) from binding with the interleukin-1 type I receptor. IL-1 causes cartilage degradation and bone resorption, worsening rheumatoid arthritis. It may cause upper respiratory tract infections and flu symptoms.

All biologicals depress the immune system, making the body more susceptible to infection. Additionally, they may prevent the immune system from properly handling cancerous cells. Injection site reactions are common with these medications.

ANTIGOUT DRUGS

The human body metabolizes purines as an everyday matter; purine metabolism produces uric acid. When uric acid concentrations exceed about 5mg/dl, it precipatates. The precipatate activates the immune system, causing pain and inflammation. Immune system responses include the secretion of IL-1B and TNF-alpha, which activates immune cells. Drugs treat gout by: 1) reducing the activation of immune cells 2) increasing the kidneys ability to excrete uric acid into the urine; 3) stopping the production of uric acid; and 4) relieving the pain and inflammation.

COLCHICINE

Colchicine decreases the ability of neutrophils to move; thus preventing them from attacking uric acid crystals, which is a source of the pain associated with gout. When neutrophils reach the uric acid crystals they release chemicals which cause inflammation, and, these chemicals also decrease the pH of the surrounding area; this lower pH, in turn, causes more uric acid to precipitate and form crystals, thus leading to the attraction of more neutrophils. Colchicine also inhibits cells from dividing by interfering with microtubules; microtubules are polymerized chains of protein assisting in the separation of DNA when cells replicate. Rapidly dividing cells such as neutrophils and gastrointestinal epithelium are affected the most.

Historically, clinicians dosed colchicine based on a patient's ability to withstand its gastrointestinal side-effects. Presently, the FDA recommends two tablets when symptoms of a gout attack appear, and, then, one additional tablet one hour later, in contrast to the traditional dosing schedule of two tablets at the first sign of an attack followed by one tablet hourly until the pain stops or diarrhea starts with a maximum of six tablets even if the pain did not stop or diarrhea did not start.

ADVERSE EFFECTS

The classical adverse effects of colchicine are diarrhea, nausea, vomiting, and abdominal pain. Additional adverse effects caused by colchicine include myelosuppression and aplastic anemia.

DRUG INTERACTIONS

In patients who have renal or hepatic impairment, colchicine is contraindicated with CYP3A4 inhibitors and/or P-gp inhibitors. In patients without renal impairment, dosages need to be adjusted for patients who are also receiving CYP3A4 inhibitors and/or P-gp inhibitors. Use caution when using colchicine with CYP3A4 inhibitors and/or P-gp inhibitors, serious adverse effects have occurred.

PROBENECID

Probenecid inhibits the reabsorption of uric acid in the proximal convoluted tubule by interfering with organic anion transporters. Essentially, probenecid stops uric acid from re-entering the blood stream once it has been secreted into fluid that will become urine.

ADVERSE EFFECTS

Probenecid may aggravate peptic ulcers, and may aggravate gout attacks when first starting, therefore, do not start probenecid until after the acute phase of a gout attack is over.

DRUG INTERACTIONS

Probenecid can increase blood levels of methotrexate. If they must be used concomitantly, lower the dose of methotrexate and monitor for adverse effects. Also, probenecid increases blood levels of penicillins, and is actually used to intentionally accomplish this in patients who require high levels of penicillins; however, avoid this combination in patients with inadequate renal function.

ALLOPURINOL

Allopurinol stops the production of uric acid by inhibiting the enzyme xanthine oxidase that makes uric acid. It may takes several weeks of therapy before allopurinol adequately lowers levels of uric acid. Allopurinol is usually dosed at 100 mg twice daily, but patients can take upto 800 mg daily in divided doses.

ADVERSE EFFECTS

Allopurinol can cause hypersensitivity reactions including vasculitis and Stevens-Johnson Syndrome. Consequently, allopurinol should be discontinued immediately if a rash develops. Allopurinol can cause hepatotoxicity, (increased alkaline phosphatase and increased liver enzymes) but it is reversible if allopurinol is stopped; consider avoiding allopurinol in patients with liver dysfunction.

DRUG INTERACTIONS

Allopurinol can increase levels of azathioprine, mercaptopurine, cyclophosphamide, carbamazepine, and vitamin K antagonists; dosage adjustments may be necessary. Conversely, antacids can decrease the absorption of allopurinol. ACE inhibitors, thiazide diuretics, and loop diuretics can increase the effects of allopurinol.

RASBURICASE

Rasburicase is a recombinant (man made) urate oxidase that metabolizes uric acid into allantoin, a substance that does not crystallize as uric acid does, and thus prevents gout attacks. Rasburicase is indicated to treat uric acid levels in patients with leukemia, lymphoma, or solid tumor malignancies on chemotherapy which is expected to cause tumor lysis, resulting in increased uric acid levels.

SIDE-EFFECTS

Severe hypersensitivity reactions have occurred, including anaphylaxis; rasburicase must be immediately and permanently discontinued in patients who develop hypersensitivity reactions. Further, rasburicase is contraindicated in patients with glucose-6-phosphate deficiency because of a risk of hemolysis.

FEBUXOSTAT

Febuxostat inhibits both forms (reduced and oxidized) of xanthine oxidase; in contrast, allopurinol only inhibits the reduced form of xanthine oxidase. Febuxostat is more effective than allopurinol at lowering serum uric acid levels.

SIDE-EFFECTS

Febuxostat has caused Stevens-Johnson Syndrome, a life-threatening hypersensitivity reaction. Also, febuxostat can adversely affect the liver; as such, liver function tests should be conducted before starting therapy. If a patient complains of symptoms indicative of liver injury then febuxostat should be stopped and liver function tests should be performed. Some may prefer to check liver function tests periodically rather than waiting for symptoms to present.

DRUG INTERACTIONS

Febuxostat is contraindicated with azathioprine and/or mercaptopurine because of increased levels of azathioprine and mercaptopurine. Febuxostat also inhibits the metabolism of theophylline.

Non-Steroidal Anti-Inflammatory Drugs				
Generic Name	Brand Name	Usual Dose	Mechanism of Action	Dosage Form
Celecoxib	Celebrex®	50-200mg twice daily as needed	Inhibits COX-2	Capsules 50 mg, 100 mg, 200 mg
Diclofenac	Voltaren®	1 twice daily	Inhibits COX-1 and COX-2	Tablets 75 mg, eye drops
Diflunisal	Dolobid	1 every 8 to 12 hours as needed	Inhibits COX-1 and COX-2	Tablets 500 mg, 1000 mg
Ibuprofen	Motrin®	1 every 6 to 8 hours as needed	Inhibits COX-1 and COX-2	Tablets: 200 mg, 400 mg, 600 mg, 800 mg. suspension, drops

Non-Steroidal Anti-Inflammatory Drugs				
Meloxicam	Mobic®	7.5 mg once to twice daily; 15 mg once daily	Same as above	Tablets 7.5 mg, 15 mg
Naproxen	Anaprox®	1 twice daily	Same as above	Tablets 250 mg, 500 mg

Disease Modifying Anti-Rheumatic Drugs: Small Molecule Drugs				
Generic Name	Brand Name	Dose	Mechanism of Action	Dosage Form
Azathioprine	Azasan® Imuran®	Adult, oral dose 1 mg/kg/day once daily or in divided doses, maximum dose of 2.5 mg/kg/day	Inhibits lymphocyte functions, thereby depressing the immune system	Tablets: 50 mg; Azasan® tablets: 75 mg and 100 mg; powder for reconstitution and injection: 100 mg vials
Cyclosporine	Gengraf® Neoral® Sandimmune®	Adult, oral dose: 2.5 mg/kg/day, divided twice daily, may increase dose by 0.5-0.75 mg/kg/day if inadequate response after 8 weeks, may increase again to maximum dose of 4 mg/kg/day	Inhibits the activation of T-lymphocytes by inhibiting the production and release of interleukin II	Neoral® capsules: 25 mg and 100 mg; Sandimmune® capsules: 25 mg and 100 mg
Hydroxychloroquine	Plaquenil®	Initial adult dose 400 mg to 600 mg daily. Usual maintenance dose is 200 mg to 400 mg daily.	Inhibits the movement of neutrophils and eosinophils thus decreasing inflammation	Tablets 200 mg
Leflunomide	Arava®	Adult initial dose: 100 mg/day for 3 days, then 10-20 mg/day	Pyrimidine-synthesis inhibitor thereby decreasing inflammation	Arava® tablets 10 mg and 20 mg
Methotrexate	Rheumatrex® Dose Pack	Adult, rheumatoid arthritis, oral dose: 7.5 mg once weekly, max of 20 mg a week	Reduces number of immune cells	Methotrexate 2.5 mg tablets; solution for injection 25 mg/ml 2 ml and 10 ml vials
Sulfasalazine	Azulfidine® Azulfidine® EN-tabs Sulfazine®	Adult, rheumatoid arthritis, oral dose: 500-1000 mg/day, increase weekly to maintenance dose of 1000mg Bid	Inhibits prostaglandin synthesis, thus decreasing inflammation	Tablet 500 mg; Delayed release tablet 500 mg

Page 112

Disease Modifying Anti-Rheumatic Drugs: Biologicals				
Generic Name Brand Name	Clinical Use	Dose	Mechanism of Action	Dosage Form
Abatacept Orencia®	Adult rheumatoid arthritis; juvenile idiopathic arthritis	Adult, IV dose for patients 60 kg to 100 kg: 750 mg for first week then 2 weeks later and then 4 weeks after initial dose, then every 4 weeks	Inhibits T cell (T lymphocyte) activation by binding to CD80 and CD86, thus preventing them from binding with CD28. This prevents full activation of T lymphocytes.	250 mg powder for reconstitution; 125 mg/ml solution in PFS
Adalimumab Humira®	Treats Rheumatoid arthritis, ankylosing spondylitis, Crohn's disease, juvenile idiopathic arthritis, plaque psoriasis, and psoriatic arthritis	Rheumatoid arthritis, psoriatic arthritis, and ankylosing spondylitis: 40 mg SubQ every other week	Adalimumab blocks tumor necrosis factor alpha (TNF-alpha) from binding with its receptor site thus preventing inflammation.	40 mg/0.8 ml prefilled pen, 40 mg/0.8 ml PFS,
Anakinra Kineret®	Treats rheumatoid arthritis in patients who have tried and failed other DMARDs	Adult, SubQ dose: 100 mg QD	IL-1 receptor antagonist, IL-1 when it binds with its receptor causes cartilage to deteriorate and causes bone resorption	Injection
Certolizumab/ Cimzia®	Reduces signs and symptoms of Crohn's disease; adult treatment of moderate to severe rheumatoid arthritis	Rheumatoid arthritis: 400 mg SubQ initially and at Weeks 2 and 4, then continue with 200 mg every other week	Binds to TNF-alpha	200 mg lyophilized powder for reconstitution, with 1 ml of sterile water for injection; 200 mg/ml prefilled syringe
Etanercept Enbrel®	Rheumatoid Arthritis	Adult: 50 mg SubQ once weekly or 25 mg subQ twice weekly	Binds to TNF-alpha	Solution for injection 50 mg/ml
Golimumab Simponi®	Moderate to severe active rheumatoid arthritis in adults when combined with MTX; active psoriatic arthritis in adults, alone or combined with MTX; active ankylosing spondylitis	All indications: 50 mg SubQ once monthly	Binds to TNF-alpha	Prefilled syringe and autoinjector each have 50 mg/0.5ml solution

Disease Modifying Anti-Rheumatic Drugs: Biologicals				
Generic Name Brand Name	Clinical Use	Dose	Mechanism of Action	Dosage Form
Infliximab Remicade®	Crohn's disease, ulcerative colitis, rheumatoid arthritis combined with methotrexate, ankylosing spondylitis, psoriatic arthritis, plaque psoriasis	Adult rheumatoid arthritis, IV dose: 3 mg/kg for the first week, 2 weeks later, and 6 weeks later, then every 6 weeks.	Binds directly to tumor necrosis factor alpha, thereby stopping TNF-alpha from binding with its receptor	100 mg of lyophilized powder in a 20 ml vial, reconstitute with 10 ml of sterile water for injection
Rituximab Rituxan®	Rheumatoid arthritis in conjunction with methotrexate	Adult rheumatoid arthritis, IV dose: 1000 mg on days 1 and 15, combined with methotrexate	Binds to the CD-20 antigen on B-lymphocytes, this activates complement-dependent cytotoxicity, meaning that biochemical steps that will kill the cell have been started.	Solution for injection: 10 mg/ml 10 ml and 50 ml vials

AntiGout Drugs				
Generic Name	Brand Name	Dose	Mechanism of Action	Dosage Form
Allopurinol	Zyloprim®	Adult dose: start at 100 mg QD, may increase to 300 mg BID for severe gout	As a xanthine oxidase inhibitor, it stops the production of uric acid	Tablets 100 mg, 300 mg
Colchicine	NA	Adult, oral, initial dose for acute attack: 0.6-1.2 mg, then 0.6 mg every 1 to 2 hours as needed, for a maximum of 6 mg or 10 tablets; wait three days before another course.	Decreases the movement of neutrophils to the urate crystals	Tablets 0.6 mg, Injection 0.5 mg/1ml 2 ml vial
Febuxostat	Uloric®	Adult dose: 40-80 mg once daily	Inhibits xanthine oxidase, thereby preventing uric acid buildup	Tablets 40 mg, 80 mg
Probenecid	NA	Adult dose: 250 mg Bid, maximum daily dose of 3 grams	Stops the kidneys from reabsorbing uric acid from urine.	Tablet 500 mg
Rasburicase	Elitek®	Pediatric dose: 0.15 mg/kg or 0.2 mg/kg once daily for 5 days; start chemotherapy 4-24 hours after the first dose	Rasburicase is an enzyme that metabolizes uric acid to allantoin, thus preventing buildup of uric acid in children with solid tumor that may lyse during chemotherapy	Injection 1.5 mg (packed with 3 one ml ampules of diluent) 7.5 mg (packed with 5 ml diluent)

Chapter 16

OPIOIDS

Opiates including morphine and its derivatives, treat a wide range of conditions including acute or chronic pain (cancer pain or otherwise), myocardial infarction, acute pulmonary edema, cough, diarrhea, and detoxification (methadone). They are used to sedate patients before surgery. Further, remifentanil, a synthetic opiate, is used to provide anesthesia during surgery.

In general, opioids work by stopping nerves from transmitting pain signals to the CNS and blocking the CNS from responding to pain signals. More specifically, opioids are agonists at opioid receptors, which include mu, delta, and kappa receptors. As agonists, opioids hyperpolarize neurons, preventing nerve signals from being sent, either to the CNS or from the CNS. Opioid receptors are found throughout the body, explaining their varied side-effects (respiratory depression, constipation, miosis, etc).

Although they have the same mechanism of action, opioids differ in their pharmacokinetic characteristics. Hydromorphone's half-life is about 2.3 hours. Codeine's half-life ranges from 2.5 to 4 hours. Morphine's half-life is 2 to 4 hours. Methadone's half-life ranges from 8 to 59 hours; it is usually dosed every 12 hours. Methadone's long duration of action makes it ideal to treat withdrawal symptoms for people addicted to opioids; its long duration of action delays withdrawal symptoms. Fentanyl's half-life, after removing a patch, ranges from 20 to 27 hours.

Morphine, an alkaloid found in the opium poppy, is widely used to treat cancer pain, myocardial infarction (the preferred drug), and chronic pain. Morphine is an agonist at the mu receptor. It can also be used for short term pain, including pain after surgery. Morphine is metabolized to several metabolites; morphine-6-glucuronide is an active metabolite. Morphine is available in immediate release tablets, extended release tablets and capsules, various strengths of oral solution, solutions for intramuscular, intravenous, or subcutaneous injection. It is also available in special preservative free solutions for epidural and intrathecal injection.

Morphine is widely used as a reference for other opiates and opioids to be compared against, particularly for dosing purposes and comparing drug structures. Many opiates are structural derivatives of morphine, including codeine. In fact, codeine is metabolized into morphine by the liver. Codeine is not a preferred drug because of the severe gastrointestinal upset that it causes some people and its relative lack of efficacy. Hydrocodone is more widely used to treat pain than codeine; although, it too can cause nausea and vomiting.

Fentanyl, a synthetic opiate, is indicated to treat moderate to severe chronic pain in opioid tolerant patients; it cannot be used in patients who have never previously used opioids. Fentanyl is not approved to be used on an as needed basis. It is an agonist at the mu receptor. Fentanyl is available as a patch, which is changed every three days. Heat sources, such as heating pads, can cause the patch to release a substantial amount of fentanyl in a shorter time frame than normal; this could cause overdose and death. CYP 3A4 inhibitors inhibit the metabolism of fentanyl; this could increase fentanyl blood levels to the point of being fatal. Fentanyl can cause fatal respiratory depression; it is contraindicated in patients with respiratory problems, including severe bronchial asthma. Fentanyl should not be used in patients with severe hepatic impairment or severe renal dysfunction.

Naloxone is an opioid antagonist used to treat acute opioid overdoses and respiratory depression, including respiratory depression in neonates. Although not FDA approved, naloxone is also used to help patients rapidly undergo detoxification. Based on its chemical structure, naloxone is probably a competitive antagonist at opioid receptors. Naloxone quickly reverses respiratory depression caused by opioid overdose. Further, when administered to a person dependent on opioids, it can cause withdrawal symptoms within minutes.

Naloxone can be administered by IV injection, IV infusion, intramuscular injection, or subcutaneous injection. Sometimes it is administered orally. For overdoses, naloxone, for adults, is dosed at 0.4 to 2 mg IV every 2 to 3 minutes as needed. If a true opiate overdose, then most patients will respond before a cumulative dose of 10 mg. Additional doses every couple of hours or a continuous intravenous infusion may be necessary to maintain adequate breathing. It can be infused at 0.0025 mg/kg hourly after an initial loading dose of 0.005 mg/kg. Additional non-pharmacological measures should be implemented to assist respiration.

For respiratory depression after surgery, naloxone is dosed at 0.1 to 0.2 mg intravenous for adults and 0.005 to 0.01 mg IV in children at 2 to 3 minute intervals.

Naltrexone, another opioid antagonist, treats alcohol dependence and helps prevent relapse in patients dependent on opioids. Naltrexone preferentially antagonizes the mu receptor.

The liver metabolizes all opioid drugs; consequently, doses need to be reduced in patients with decreased liver function to prevent adverse effects resulting from greater bioavailability. Morphine and codeine are both metabolized by the liver to morphine-6-glucuronide.

Decreased kidney function lowers clearance, and, therefore, increases blood levels of morphine, codeine, meperidine, and their metabolites. Further, meperidine, a drug known to cause seizures, and its metabolite nor-meperidine may build up in the blood when the kidneys are not functioning well, thus exposing the patient to an increased risk of seizures.

SIDE-EFFECTS

Opioids produce many different adverse effects. Minor adverse effects include nausea, vomiting, dizziness, constipation, miosis (pupil constriction), somnolence, and mental lethargy. Severe adverse effects include respiratory depression, dysphoria, anaphylactic reactions, and hypotension. Because of CNS effects and miosis use caution when using opiates in patients with head injuries. Opioid use in a patient with a head injury makes it difficult to determine whether miosis is due to the head injury or opioid use. Further, opioids increase intracranial pressure, which may aggravate intracranial pressure resulting from a head injury.

Opioids may strongly decrease respiration by directly affecting the brainstem's respiratory neurons. Opioids reduce the brainstem's response to carbon dioxide levels. Opioid induced respiratory depression can occur in any patient, however, elderly patients and patients with a respiratory problems are at particular risk. Clinicians should use other strategies for pain management before using opioids in these patients. If opioids are used, as with all drugs, the lowest possible dose should be used.

DRUG INTERACTIONS

Opioids interact with drugs from other classes and alcohol. The concurrent use of opioids and other drugs having CNS side-effects can amplify the side-effects experienced by the patient. For example, morphine co-administered with a benzodiazepine increases the sedation a patient experiences and can be fatal. Also, alcohol can inhibit morphine metabolism, potentially causing death. Furthermore, muscle relaxants combined with opioids have a synergistic influence on decreasing respiration.

OPIOIDS				
Generic Name	Brand Name	Clinical Use	Adult Dose	Dosage Form
APAP/codeine	Tylenol/Codeine #3® and Tylenol®/ Codeine #4	Moderate to severe pain	1/2 to 2 tablets every 4 to 6 hours as needed	Tylenol/Codeine #3® and generic tablets 300 mg/30mg Tylenol®/Codeine #4 and generic tablets 300 mg/60mg
Butorphanol	NA	Moderate to severe pain; post- operative pain; migraine headache	Post- operative pain: 1-4 mg IM or 0.5-2 mg IV every 3 to 4 hours	Vials 1 mg/ml vials and 2 mg/ml vials. Nasal spray 10 mg/ml
Codeine Sulfate	NA	Mild to moderate pain	15 mg to 60 mg every 4 to 6 hours as needed. Take with food.	Tablets 15 mg, 30 mg, 60 mg

OPIOIDS

Generic Name	Brand Name	Clinical Use	Adult Dose	Dosage Form
Fentanyl	Duragesic®	Severe Pain	1 Patch of any strength applied topically every 72 hours	Brand and generic patches all in mcg/hour: 12, 25, 50, 75 100.
Hydrocodone/ Acetamino- phen	Vicodin® Norco®	Moderate to severe pain	1 to 2 tablets every 4 to 6 hours as needed for pain.	Tablet 5 mg hydrocodone and 300 mg acetaminophen
Hydromor- phone	Dilaudid®	Moderate to severe pain	1-2 Q6H PRN PAIN	Brand and generic tablets 2 mg, 4 mg, 8 mg; Vials 1mg/1ml
Levorphanol	Levo-Dromoran	Moderate to severe pain; chronic pain caused by can- cer	Adult initial dose for severe pain: 4 mg every 6 to 8 hours as needed, maintenance dose: titrate dose by 8 mg daily every 3-5 days	Brand and generic tablets 2 mg
Meperidine	Demerol®	Moderate to severe pain	Adult dose: 50 mg to 150 mg every 3 to 4 hours as needed	Brand and generic tablets 50 mg, 100 mg; vials 10 mg/ml
Methadone	Dolophine®	Moderate to severe pain; de- toxification and maintenance as part of an FDA program	Adult pain dose 5 mg mg to 10 mg every 8 to 12 hours as needed for pain	Brand and generic tablets 5mg and 10 mg
Morphine	Avinza®, Kadi- an®, MS Contin®, Roxanol®	Moderate to severe acute and chronic pain	Adult dose immediate release tablets: 10 mg every 4 hours as need- ed, maintenance dose: highly individualized	MS Contin® brand and generic tablets 15 mg, 30 mg, 60 mg, 100 mg, 200 mg. MS Contin is extended release
Oxycodone/ac- etaminophen	Percocet® Tylox®	Moderate to Severe pain	1 to 2 tablets every 4 to 6 hours as needed for pain.	Percocet® and generic tab- lets all in mg: 2.5/325, 5/325, 7.5/325, 7.5/500, 10/325, 10/650

OPIOIDS				
Generic Name	Brand Name	Clinical Use	Adult Dose	Dosage Form
Oxycodone	Oxycontin®	Moderate to severe pain	Dose for Oxycontin®: starting dose should be 10 mg every 12 hours for patients who have not had prior opiate therapy. Use conversion guidelines in package insert for patients switching from another opiate.	Oxycontin® 10 mg, 15 mg, 20 mg, 30 mg, 40 mg, 60 mg, 80 mg. Oxycontin® is an extended release formulation of oxycodone. Oxycodone generic tablets: 5 mg, 10 mg, 15 mg, 20 mg, 30 mg. Oral solution 20 mg/ml
Pentazocine	Talwin®	Moderate to severe pain	Adult IM or SubQ: 30-60 mg every 3 to 4 hours, max dose of 60 mg at a time, max dose of 360 mg in 24 hours	Vials 30 mg/ml
Tramadol	Ultram® Ultram® ER	Moderate to moderately-severe pain	50 mg to 100 mg every 6 hours as needed for pain	Brand and generic tablets 50 mg immediate release and 100 mg, 200 mg, 300 mg extended release

CHAPTER 17

GASTROINTESTINAL DRUGS

Acid Protecting Drugs		
Proton Pump Inhibitors	Histamine (H$_2$) Blockers	Miscellaneous
Omeprazole Lansoprazole Esomeprazole Pantoprazole Rabeprazole	Cimetidine Famotidine Nizantidine Ranitidine	Sucralfate Metoclopramide Misoprostol

Histamine (H$_2$) blockers prevent histamine from binding with its receptors in stomach parietal cells, which is a necessary step for the production of stomach acid. H$_2$ blockers are well tolerated and still used by many patients. Cimetidine, an H$_2$ blocker, inhibits the metabolism of many drugs; therefore it is important to question patients about their use of cimetidine. Cimetidine is available over the counter.

Proton pump inhibitors are much stronger than H$_2$ blockers. Each is generally as effective as the other. Omeprazole inhibits CYP 2C19; in particular, it prevents the activation of clopidogrel (anti-clotting agent) to its active form. Omeprazole and lansoprazole are available over the counter. Question patients about their use of OTC omeprazole.

Sucralfate forms a protective coating over ulcers in the stomach, preventing stomach acid from further attacking ulcers, providing time to heal. Other medications need to be spaced from sucralfate by at least two hours.

Misoprostol is a prostaglandin replacement. Prostaglandins protect the stomach lining from stomach acid, preventing ulcer formation.

Ulcers can form in the stomach and/or duodenum (the first part of the small intestine, connected to the stomach). Ulcers are caused by the bacteria, H. Pylori, but may also form, without H. Pylori, by excess stomach acid or NSAIDs, or the cause may be unknown. Physicians treat ulcers caused by H. Pylori with a combination of acid reducing agents and antibiotics. Prevpac®, a combination of lansoprazole, amoxicillin, and clarithromycin, treats ulcers caused by H. Pylori.

To help prevent ulcers caused by NSAIDs, misoprostol, a prostaglandin, is combined with NSAIDs to replace the prostaglandins that NSAIDs prevent from being formed. In fact, the drug Arthrotec™ is a combination of diclofenac and misoprostol in one tablet. Alcohol also decreases prostaglandin production, which is why people who regularly consume alcohol often have ulcers.

GERD

Gastroesophageal Reflux Disease (GERD) is when stomach acid and digested food move upwards back into the esophagus. GERD is also known as heartburn. Left untreated, severe GERD can cause esophageal cancer. GERD treatment depends on the stage (I, II, or III) of GERD. Stage I, entailing sporadic symptoms, can be treated with lifestyle modifications, weight loss, antacids, and histamine H2 receptor blockers. Stage II, which entails frequent symptoms, is treated with proton pump inhibitors; some clinicians recommend uninterrupted treatment and others recommend treatment only when symptoms are active. Stage III, entailing chronic non-stop symptoms, is treated with uninterrupted proton pump inhibitors dosed at least once daily and sometimes twice daily.

IRRITABLE BOWEL SYNDROME

Patients with Irritable Bowel Syndrome (IBS) report abdominal pain, diarrhea, and or constipation. Treatment focuses on reducing symptoms primarily because the exact cause is unknown. Fiber treats both diarrhea and constipation; in diarrhea, it absorbs extra water; in constipation, it pulls water in, easing stool passage. Dicyclomine treats the pain associated with cramping. Lubiprostone helps reduce constipation. Diphenoxylate with atropine treats diarrhea associated with IBS.

CONSTIPATION

Constipation, a common ailment, often results from a lack of fiber. Modern medicine uses old-time remedies to promote bowel movements. Fiber, found in abundance in many foods, but lacking in most diets, bulks and lubricates stool. Lubricants also promote the passage of stool.

DIARRHEA

Diarrhea generally results from the introduction of foreign bacteria to the GI tract, overgrowth of naturally occurring bacteria, excess magnesium, drugs, or other possible causes. Diarrhea caused by antibiotic use is sometimes treated with other antibiotics, such as, metronidazole. Severe diarrhea necessitates IV fluids, especially so in the young and elderly.

DRUGS

PROTON PUMP INHIBITORS

Proton pump inhibitors (PPIs) include dexlansoprazole, esomeprazole, lansoprazole, omeprazole, pantoprazole, and rabeprazole. PPIs treat ulcers and GERD; they can be used acutely or long-term. These drugs inhibit the H^+- K^+-ATPase-pump that pumps acid (H^+) into the stomach. All are equally effective at reducing stomach acid by 80-90%. Stomach acid can physically destroy these drugs, and, consequently, the various dosage forms are formulated to allow them to pass through the stomach without being inactivated. These drugs do not work in the stomach, but rather work inside the stomach wall, and, consequently, must be absorbed in the intestinal tract and then distributed to the stomach wall by blood flow. Despite the protective dosage forms, increased stomach acid occurring when eating food can be strong enough to overcome the dosage formulation, as a result, these drugs should be administered at least 30 minutes before food or two hours after food.

SIDE-EFFECTS

Proton pump inhibitors are well tolerated. Most side-effects are limited to nausea, vomiting, constipation, or diarrhea; all of which occur infrequently. Proton pump inhibitors may cause vitamin B12 deficiency when used for more than a few months. The body normally has a substantial store of vitamin B12, so short-term use does not cause vitamin B12 deficiency.

DRUG INTERACTIONS

Omeprazole inhibits CYP2C19. CYP2C19 converts the prodrug clopidogrel (an anti-clotting drug) to its active form. Omeprazole can prevent the conversion of clopidogrel to its active form, thus leaving the patient at risk of clotting. Another proton pump inhibitor should be substituted for omeprazole in this situation. Omeprazole may induce CYP1A2. CYP1A2 metabolizes several drugs including theophylline (a treatment for asthma).

HISTAMINE BLOCKERS

Histamine receptor antagonists (H_2 blockers) block histamine from binding with its receptor in stomach parietal cells, which is a necessary step for the production of stomach acid. Histamine receptor antagonists are well tolerated, and it is rare to discontinue one of these because of side-effects. In contrast to proton pump inhibitors, food may increase absorption of H2 antagonists. Plasma protein binding is insignificant. Reducing the dose is generally unnecessary for patients with liver dysfunction. Decrease doses for patients with decreased creatinine clearance.

SIDE-EFFECTS

Most side-effects are limited to nausea, vomiting, constipation, and muscle fatigue, which occur infrequently. Cimetidine interferes with testosterone, leading to side-effects such as gynecomastia.

DRUG INTERACTIONS

Cimetidine inhibits CYP1A2, CYP2C9, and CYP2D6, increasing blood levels of drugs metabolized by these enzymes. Despite proton pump inhibitors largely displacing cimetidine, many older patients continue to use cimetidine (over the counter) because they are hesitant to switch medications once they find something that works. The other histamine receptor antagonists, such as ranitidine and famotidine, do not significantly interact with CYP isoenzymes.

OTHER ACID PROTECTING DRUGS

Sucralfate

Sucralfate adheres to ulcers, protecting the ulcer from acid and other digestive enzymes that would otherwise make it very difficult for the ulcer to heal. Sucralfate is indicated for both short-term and maintenance therapy of duodenal ulcers. Sucralfate is well tolerated. It should be administered one hour before meals and at bedtime.

SIDE-EFFECTS

Sucralfate contains aluminum, which is excreted by the kidneys. Use sucralfate with caution, if at all, in patients with chronic renal failure. Excess aluminum can cause osteodystrophy, osteomalacia, and encephalopathy.

DRUG INTERACTIONS

Sucralfate's affect on warfarin therapy varies from patient to patient; monitor therapy closely; suggest separating them by two hours. Sucralfate reduces the absorption of digoxin, fluoroquinolone antibiotics, ketoconazole, levothyroxine, phenytoin, quinidine, ranitidine, tetracycline, and theophylline. These drugs should be taken two hours before sucralfate to allow them time to absorb.

Misoprostol

Misoprostol, a prostaglandin, reduces the risk of NSAID induced gastric ulcers (it has not been shown to help with duodenal ulcers). It reduces stomach acid secretion, and increases bicarbonate and mucus production, all three of which protect the stomach. NSAIDs prevent the formation of stomach-protective prostaglandins. Misoprostol is available alone or in combination with the NSAID diclofenac.

SIDE-EFFECTS

Misoprostol can cause serious or fatal harm to unborn babies- avoid use in pregnant women.

DRUG INTERACTIONS

Misoprostol should not be used within four hours of oxytocic drugs. Misoprostol and magnesium together may cause diarrhea.

Metoclopramide

Metoclopramide is approved for the short-term treatment of GERD in patients who have tried conventional therapy. It is also approved to treat diabetic gastric stasis. Metoclopramide works by sensitizing tissues to acetylcholine. Acetylcholine stimulates gastrointestinal motility.

SIDE-EFFECTS

Metoclopramide may cause tardive dyskinesia, a serious movement disorder producing movements similiar to Parkinson's Disease, and is often irreversible, possibly necessitating permanent drug therapy. Metoclopramide may increase the frequency and severity of seizures and should be avoided in patients with epilepsy. Further, it may cause mental depression; use in patients with a history of mental depression only if the benefits outweigh the risks. It may cause, rarely, neuroleptic malignant syndrome (NMS), a potentially fatal syndrome manifesting as hyperthermia, muscle rigidity, altered consciousness, altered cardiovascular function, and excessive sweating (diaphoresis).

Do not use metoclopramide during gastrointestinal hemorrhage, mechanical obstruction, or when part of the GI tract is perforated.

DRUG INTERACTIONS

Since metoclopramide works by sensitizing tissues to acetylcholine, anticholinergic drugs naturally reduce the effectiveness of metoclopramide. Further, opioids antagonize the effectiveness of metoclopramide; opioids decrease gastrointestinal motility. Avoid use in patients using monoamine oxidase inhibitors because of the possibility of increased blood pressure in patients who already have hypertension.

Chloride Channel Activator

Lubiprostone is indicated for both chronic idiopathic constipation and irritable bowel syndrome with constipation. It causes intestinal chloride channels to secrete a chloride-rich fluid into the intestinal tract, increasing intestinal motility and the passing of stool, all while minimizing the symptoms of irritable bowel syndrome. Patients should be examined for a mechanical obstruction before starting lubiprostone.

SIDE-EFFECTS

Nausea, diarrhea, headache, abdominal pain, abdominal distension, and gas are the most common side-effects of lubiprostone. Dyspnea may occur within an hour of the first dose, and usually resolves within three hours; some patients experience dyspnea upon repeat dosing; some patients may decide to discontinue use.

DRUG INTERACTIONS

Lubiprostone is not metabolized by the liver. Further, lubiprostone does not have any known plasma protein interactions.

Serotonin Agonists

Tegaserod is a partial agonist at $5\text{-}HT_4$ receptors (subtype of serotonin receptors) in the gastrointestinal tract. Tegaserod returns intestinal motility to a normal state throughout the GI tract. Tegaserod treats irritable bowel syndrome in women patients suffering mainly from constipation. It also treats chronic idiopathic constipation in patients younger than 65.

SIDE-EFFECTS

Tegaserod sometimes causes severe diarrhea that may require discontinuing the drug. Severe diarrhea may cause hypotension and/or syncope. Discontinue tegaserod if abrupt abdominal pain occurs. Discontinue tegaserod if ischemic colitis symptoms occur.

DRUG INTERACTIONS

Tegaserod does not interfere with the metabolism of dextromethorphan, a known substrate of CYP 2D6; therefore, it is not expected to interfere with other substrates of CYP2D6. Additionally, tegaserod does not affect theophylline's metabolism, a CYP1A2 substrate. Tegaserod does not significantly affect digoxin levels. Tegaserod does not affect warfarin pharmacokinetics or pharmacodynamics. Tegaserod should not interfere with oral contraceptives.

Proton Pump Inhibitors - GERD, Ulcers			
Generic Name	Brand Name	Dose	Dosage Form
Esomeprazole	Nexium®	20 mg to 40 mg once to twice daily	Capsules, Granules, Injection
Lansoprazole	Prevacid®	20 mg to 40 mg once to twice daily	Tablets orally disintegrating, Capsules, Granules, Injection
Omeprazole	Prilosec®	20 mg to 40 mg once to twice daily	Tablet 20 mg, Capsule 20 mg
Pantoprazole	Protonix®	20 mg to 40 mg once daily	Tablets 20 mg and 40 mg, Injection
Rabeprazole	Aciphex®	20 mg to 40 mg once to twice daily	Tablets 20 mg

Histamine Receptor Blockers (H_2 Blockers) - GERD, Ulcers

Generic Name	Brand Name	Dose	Dosage Form
Cimetidine	Tagamet®	Adult dose 300 mg four times daily	Tablet 300 mg
Famotidine	Pepcid®	Adult 40 mg at bedtime	Tablet, Chewable tablet, Powder for oral suspension, Injection
Nizantidine	Axid®	Adult 150 mg twice daily or 300 mg at bedtime	Tablet 75 mg, Capsule 150 mg, 300 mg, Oral solution 15 mg/ml
Ranitidine	Zantac®	Adult 150 mg twice daily	Tablets 75 mg, 150 mg, 300 mg, Capsules 150 mg, 300 mg, Syrup 15 mg/ml, Injection 25 mg/ml

Other Drugs Protecting the Stomach from Acid (GERD / Ulcers)

Generic Name	Brand Name	Dose	Mechanism of Action	Dosage Form
Metoclopramide	Reglan®	Adults 10-15 mg upto four times daily	Enhances the body's response to acetylcholine thus enhancing motility and accelerating gastric emptying. Treats GERD	Tablets 5 mg, 10 mg
Misoprostol	Cytotec®	Adults 200 mcg four times daily, reduce dose if not well tolerated	Replaces protective prostaglandins that NSAIDs prevent from being formed	Tablets 100 mcg, 200 mcg
Sucralfate	Carafate®	Adult 1 gm every 4 hours	Forms a protective coating over ulcers, promoting healing	Tablets 1 gram, Suspension 1 gm/10ml

Antidiarrheals

Generic Name	Brand Name	Dose	Mechanism of Action	Dosage Form
Cholestyramine	Questran®	4 grams of powder up to 6 times in 24 hours	Bile salts can cause diarrhea, Cholestyramine binds bile salts, thus preventing diarrhea	Powder Packs of 4 grams each or available in a can with powder and a scoop
Diphenoxylate with Atropine	Lomotil®, Lonox	Adults 5 mg four times daily (maximum of 20 mg/day), then reduce dose	Diphenoxylate, an opioid agonist, slows GI motility; Atropine, and anticholinergic also slow motility	Tablet 2.5 mg of diphenoxylate and 0.025mg of atropine, Oral solution
Loperamide	Imodium®	Adults acute: 4 mg initially, then 2 mg after each loose stool, max of 16 mg/24hours	Opioid derivative, slows GI motility	Tablet 2mg, Capsule 2mg, Oral Solution 1mg/5ml

Irritable Bowel Syndrome				
Generic Name	Brand Name	Dose	Mechanism of Action	Dosage Form
Desipramine	Norpramin®	Adults 10 mg at bedtime	Decrease pain from IBS	Tablet 10 mg, 25 mg, 50 mg, 75 mg, 100 mg, 150 mg
Dicyclomine	Bentyl®	Adult oral dose initiate with 20 mg four times daily then increase to 160 mg/day if needed	Reduces cramping	Tablet 20 mg, Capsule 10 mg, Syrup 10 mg/5ml, Injection 10 mg/ml
Lubiprostone	Amitiza®	Adults 8 mcg twice daily	Reduces constipation	Capsules: 8 mcg and 24 mcg
Polyethylene Glycol	Miralax®	Adult 17 gm mixed in 8 ounces of water	Reduces constipation	Powder
Tegaserod	Zelnorm®	Adults IBS with constipation 6 mg twice daily before meals for 4-6 weeks	As a partial serotonin agonist, it stimulates peristalsis, thus correcting constipation	Tablets 2 mg, 6 mg

Ulcerative Colitis				
Generic Name	Brand Name	Dose	Mechanism of Action	Dosage Form
Balsalazide	Colazal®	Adults 2.25 gms three times daily	Body converts it to mesalamine, decreases inflammatory response	Capsule 750 mg
Olsalazine	Dipentum®	Adults 500 mg twice daily	Decreases the body's inflammatory response	Capsule 250 mg
Mesalamine	Asacol®, Asacol® 800, Canasa®, Pentasa®, Rowasa®, Lialda®	Adults 1 gm orally four times daily	Decreases the inflammatory response	Asacol® tablet 400 mg, Lialda® 1.2 gm, Pentasa® Capsule 250 mg, 500 mg, Canasa® Suppository 1000 mg, Rowasa® Rectal Suspension 4 gm/60ml
Prednisone	Deltasone®	Adult dose varies considerably from patient to patient	Decreases the inflammatory response	Tablets 2.5 mg, 5 mg, 10 mg, 20 mg, 50mg
Sulfasalazine	Azulfidine®, Azulfidine EN® Tabs	Adult initial 1 gram 3 to 4 times daily, maintenance dose 2 gm/day	Decreases the inflammatory response, systemically inhibits prostaglandin synthesis	Tablet 500 mg, Tablet delayed release 500 mg

CHAPTER 18

RESPIRATORY AND NASAL DRUGS

BRONCHODILATORS	ANTI-INFLAMMATORIES		MUCOLYTICS
Beta agonists: Albuterol Metaproterenol Pirbuterol Levalbuterol Salmeterol **Anticholinergics:** Ipratropium Tiotropium **Methylxanthines:** Theophylline	**Corticosteroids:** Beclomethasone Budesonide Flunisolide Fluticasone Mometasone Prednisone **Mast Cell Inhibitors:** Cromolyn Nedocromil	**Leukotriene Receptor Antagonists:** Montelukast Zafirlukast	Acetylcysteine Dornase Alfa

Respiratory problems generally result from an overactive immune response. Respiratory medications decrease the chronic inflammation, constricted bronchioles, and plugged airways commonly found in patients with asthma, COPD, and cystic fibrosis. Bronchodilators include beta agonists, anticholinergics, and methylxanthines. Beta agonists stimulate beta receptors, increasing intracellular cAMP levels, thus dilating bronchioles, increasing air flow into the lungs. Anticholinergics compete with acetylcholine for binding at muscarinic receptors, thus decreasing mucus production, thus dilating airways, allowing for easier breathing. Methylxanthines increase cAMP levels, ultimately dilating bronchioles.

Corticosteroids, acting by several different means, prevent immune cells from producing inflammatory factors which inflame and block airways. Further, corticosteroids promote the production of factors that decrease inflammation. Mast cell inhibitors stabilize mast cells, (immune cells responsible for releasing inflammatory chemicals) preventing them from releasing their inflammatory contents.

Leukotriene receptor antagonists block leukotrienes from binding with their receptors in the lungs. Leukotrienes swell and inflame airways. Zileuton prevents the production of leukotrienes.

Acetylcysteine breaks mucus apart; its free sulfhydryl group breaks the disulfide bonds in mucus, decreasing its viscosity, allowing the lungs to more easily remove it. Dornase Alfa cleaves the excess strands of DNA in cystic fibrosis, allowing the excess DNA laden mucus to be more easily removed from the lungs.

ASTHMA

Chronically inflamed lungs characterize both asthma and chronic obstructive pulmonary disease (COPD). Many different immune cells cause inflammation in respiratory diseases. Different cells and mediators inflame the lungs in asthma than in COPD. In asthma, lymphocytes, mast cells, and eosinophils cause considerable inflammation. In asthma, allergens stimulate mast cells to release: 1) bradykinin, 2) eosinophilic chemotactic factor, 3) histamine, and 4) leukotrienes.

These substances swell the walls of small bronchioles. They also cause bronchioles to secrete airway-clogging mucus; and they constrict larger bronchioles, making breathing difficult in asthmatics.

Asthma medications dilate bronchioles and decrease the immune response. Albuterol, and other beta-agonists, usually effectively dilate bronchioles, allowing easier breathing. Long-term use of inhaled corticosteroids decreases chronic inflammation, lessening the need to use albuterol or other rescue inhalers.

COPD

Chronic Obstructive Pulmonary Disease (COPD), includes emphysema and chronic bronchitis. In COPD, macrophages are activated by allergens, such as cigarette smoke or smog. Macrophages then activate neutrophils, T-lymphocytes, and monocytes. Neutrophils release proteases, causing two of the three main problems associated with COPD. First, proteases destroy alveolar cell walls. This slow but eventual destruction makes it difficult to expel air, resulting in air being trapped in the lungs. Second, proteases cause hyper-secretion of mucus, blocking airways. Third, macrophages also activate fibroblasts, resulting in fibrosis of small airways, further making it difficult to expel air.

Bronchodilators, such as albuterol, ease breathing for patients with COPD. Anticholinergics, such as ipratropium or tiotropium, block muscarinic receptors, preventing acetylcholine induced bronchoconstriction, thus relaxing and dilating bronchioles. Anticholinergics are preferred over beta agonists because they have less cardiac side-effects. Oral or nebulized corticosteroids reduce the symptoms of acute COPD episodes. Nebulized steroids have less systemic side-effects than oral steroids have.

CYSTIC FIBROSIS

Cystic fibrosis, a genetic disorder, involves neutrophils producing excess polymerized DNA that forms abnormally thick mucus. Innumerable strands of polymerized DNA form the excess mucus. This mucus particularly affects the lungs. Lung infections are common because the lungs have a difficult time clearing the thick mucus. Tobramycin is used to treat these infections.

Until recently, drug therapy was limited to breaking down the thick mucus to help the body remove it better. As a DNA enzyme, dornase Alfa breaks down the mucus once it has formed. Dornase Alfa selectively cleaves the extracellular DNA that forms the mucus. Dornase Alfa is a biotechnology drug. Once these bonds are broken, the mucus becomes less thick and the body can remove it more easily. Dornase Alfa is dosed once daily via a nebulizer. Its adverse-effects include chest pain, fever, throat irritation, runny nose, and an altered voice.

Presently, ivacaftor is the only drug that decreases the production of abnormally thick mucus. Ivacaftor improves the function of a defective protein that causes cystic fibrosis.

DRUGS

BETA AGONISTS

Beta-2 selective agonists are used for asthma and COPD. Generally stated, beta-agonists bind with beta-2 receptors on airway smooth muscle, relaxing and opening the airways. Specifically, upon binding, beta-agonists increase levels of cyclic adenosine monophosphate (cAMP), which in turn increases levels of protein kinase A (PKA). PKA, in turn, activates potassium (K^+) channels; inhibits phospholipase C; inhibits activation of myosin light chain kinase; activates myosin light chain phosphatase; and decreases intracellular calcium either by moving it out of the cells or into storage vesicles inside the cell. All of these events relax airway smooth muscle, allowing easier breathing.

Short-acting beta agonists include albuterol, metaproterenol, pirbuterol, and levalbuterol. Short-acting beta agonists may need to be dosed once to four times daily. They can be used on an as-needed basis or on a scheduled basis. Salmeterol is a long-acting beta agonist that only needs twice daily dosing.

SIDE-EFFECTS

Overall, beta-agonists produce few untolerable side-effects. Beta-agonists used to treat asthma are primarily beta-2 selective; however, they may increase heart rate and blood pressure. Some people experience an uncomfortably rapid heart rate; these patients should try levalbuterol, which least affects the heart. Other side-effects include muscle tremor and hypokalemia; arrhythmias from hypokalemia are quite rare.

DRUG INTERACTIONS

Monoamine oxidase inhibitors prevent the metabolism of orally administered albuterol.

ANTICHOLINERGICS

Ipratropium and tiotropium block acetylcholine from binding with muscarinic receptors, thus dilating bronchioles; acetylcholine normally causes bronchoconstriction. Ipratropium is used three to four times daily. Tiotropium, dosed once daily, is a capsule, the contents of which are inhaled with the use of an inhaler; a patient should inhale twice for each capsule to ensure the entire dose was inhaled. For asthmatic patients, add an anticholinergic drug after a long acting beta agonist has failed to provide adequate relief or a beta-agonist causes unacceptable side-effects, such as tremor. In asthmatic patients, beta-agonists are more effective at dilating bronchioles than anticholinergics. In contrast, patients with COPD respond better to an anticholinergic than a beta-agonist. These drugs do not significantly interact with other drugs because they are not significantly systemically absorbed.

SIDE-EFFECTS

Tiotropium is associated with upper respiratory tract infections in 41% of patients. Ipratropium is associated with upper respiratory tract infections in 9-34% of patients. Tiotropium may cause dry mouth in about 15% of patients. Inhaled ipratropium is known to have a bitter taste sometimes limiting compliance; whereas nebulized ipratropium does not have this problem.

METHYLXANTHINES

At high doses, theophylline dilates bronchioles by blocking phosphodiesterase, which results in increased intracellular levels of cAMP. Increased cAMP levels dilate bronchioles. Theophylline also decreases the number of eosinophils; and it decreases the production of inflammatory factors in immune cells by decreasing the activity of genes responsible for producing inflammatory factors. This latter benefit can be achieved at low doses, preventing side-effects.

Theophylline, similar in structure to caffeine, stimulates the heart, possibly causing increased heart rate or heart flutter. These cardiovascular side-effects cause theophylline to be a last choice drug for asthma or COPD. Theophylline is primarily used in severe asthma or COPD patients when beta-agonists and corticosteroids are not adequately treating the patient.

DRUG INTERACTIONS

Theophylline may increase heart rate and blood pressure; when given with other stimulatory drugs, these effects may be additive or synergistic.

CORTICOSTEROIDS

Corticosteroids are widely used for asthma and occasionally used for COPD. Corticosteroids prevent immune cells from producing inflammatory factors, which inflame and block airways; further, corticosteroids promote the production of factors that decrease inflammation. In asthma, T-lymphocytes and mast cells release inflammatory-factors that inflame air passages. In these cells, corticosteroids bind with the glucocorticoid-receptor to form a complex; the complex of drug and receptor then enters the cell nucleus and prevents the DNA of these cells from directing the production of these inflammatory-factors; also, as opposed to binding with DNA or genes, the complex of drug and receptor prevents the production of inflammatory-factors by binding with protein transcription factors.

Inhaled corticosteroids include fluticasone propionate (Flovent®), beclomethasone dipropionate (QVAR®), and budesonide (Pulmicort Flexhaler®). Oral corticosteroids for asthma and COPD include prednisone tablets, methylprednisolone tablets, prednisolone solution, and dexamethasone tablets.

Start using inhaled corticosteroids in mild asthma, the second level of severity of asthma classifications.

SIDE-EFFECTS

Inhaled corticosteroids, as a class, are not absorbed well systemically, and, therefore have limited systemic side-effects. However, beclomethasone diprionate is absorbed systemically. Beclomethasone can suppress the hypothalamic-pituitary-adrenal axis (HPA) at doses of 2000 micrograms daily. Prednisone, an orally administered corticosteroid, suppresses the HPA axis at doses of 7.5 mg daily or higher. Inhaled corticosteroids may cause throat irritation in some patients; rinsing with water is helpful.

Side-effects associated with long-term use of orally administered corticosteroids include cataracts, diabetes, fluid retention, osteoporosis, peptic ulcers, psychosis, thinning of the skin, and weight gain.

DRUG INTERACTIONS

Inhaled corticosteroids do not have any substantial drug interactions because they are not well absorbed.

NASAL ALLERGIES

Allergens can cause nasal inflammation. Corticosteroids, when sprayed, into the nose, decrease the release of inflammatory factors responsible for nasal drainage. Further, anticholinergics, (ipratropium nasal solution) also decrease nasal drainage. Antihistamines block histamine from reaching its receptor, thus preventing the formation of nasal drainage. Lipophilic antihistamines enter the brain and cause drowsiness. Histamine plays a role in keeping the brain awake. Ionized antihistamines (fexofenadine, loratadine, cetirizine) do not enter the brain because they are not lipophilic, and, therefore, do not cause drowsiness. The older antihistamines such as diphenhydramine and chlorpheniramine enter the brain and cause drowsiness. Aside from drowsiness, antihistamines cause few substantial side-effects.

Bronchodilators: Beta Agonists

Generic Name	Brand Name	Dose	Mechanism of Action	Dosage Form
Albuterol	Proventil® Ventolin®	2 Puffs 2 to 4 times daily as needed	Activates beta$_2$ receptors causing bronchodilation	Tablets 2 mg, 4 mg, Inhaler 90 mcg/inhalation, Syrup 2 mg/5ml, Aerosol for nebulization
Levalbuterol	Xopenex®	2 Puffs every 4 to 6 hours as needed	Same as above	Inhaler and Aerosol for nebulization
Metaproterenol	Alupent®	2-3 inhalations every 3 to 4 hours as needed	Same as above	Tablets 10 mg, 20 mg, Syrup 10 mg/5ml, Aerosol 0.65 mg/inhalation
Pirbuterol	Maxair® Autohaler	2 Inhalations every 4 to 6 hours as needed	Same as above	Inhaler
Salmeterol	Serevent®	One inhalation twice daily	Long acting beta$_2$ receptor agonist, relaxes bronchial smooth muscles	Powder for inhalation, inhaler

Bronchodilators: Anticholinergics

Generic Name	Brand Name	Dose	Mechanism of Action	Dosage Form
Ipratropium	Atrovent®	COPD / asthma 2 puffs orally 4 times daily, max 12 inhalations/24hours (asthma); Nasal allergies: 2 sprays each nostril 2 to 3 times daily	Blocks acetylcholine, decreases secretions, dilates bronchioles	Atrovent HFA Inhaler 17 mcg/spray (asthma); Solution for nebulization 0.02% (asthma); Atrovent Nasal Spray 0.03%, 0.06%, 15ml
Tiotropium	Spiriva®	Inhale 1 capsule once daily with inhaler	Same as above	Capsule 18 mcg for inhalation

Bronchodilators: Methylxanthines

Theophylline	Theo-24®	Adult maintenance dose: 400 mg -600 mg daily	Dilates bronchioles	Theo-24 capsules: 100 mg, 200 mg, 300 mg

Corticosteroids

Generic Name	Brand Name	Dose	Mechanism of Action	Dosage Form
Beclomethasone	QVAR®	1-2 puffs twice daily	Decreases production of inflammatory factors	Inhaler 40 mcg and 80 mcg
Budesonide	Pulmicort Flex-haler®	2 puffs twice daily	Same as above	Inhaler 90 mcg, 180mcg, 200mcg
Flunisolide	Aerobid®	2 puffs twice daily upto 8 puffs/24hours maximum	Same as above	Aerobid 250 mcg/ spray
Fluticasone	Flovent® HFA	2 puffs twice daily	Same as above	Inhaler 44 mcg, 110 mcg, 220 mcg
Mometasone	Asmanex®	1-2 puffs once daily	Same as above	Inhaler 220 mcg
Prednisone	Deltasone®	Many different doses. 6 day taper starting at 60 mg and decreasing by 10 mg daily for 6 days.	Same as above	Tablets 2.5 mg, 5 mg, 10 mg, 20 mg, 50mg

Mast Cell Stabilizers

Generic Name	Brand Name	Dose	Mechanism of Action	Dosage Form
Cromolyn	NasalCrom®	1 spray each nostril 3 to 4 times daily	Stops mast cells from releasing histamine, histamine causes inflammation.	NasalCrom® 40mg/ ml
Nedocromil	Alocril®	1 to 2 drops in affected eye(s) twice daily	Inhibits inflammatory cells such as eosinophils, neutrophils, macrophages, and mast cells.	Opthalmic solution 2%

Leukotriene-Receptor Antagonists

Generic Name	Brand Name	Dose	Mechanism of Action	Dosage Form
Montelukast	Singulair®	Adult 10 mg once daily	Blocks the receptor for leukotrienes.	Tablets 4 mg chewable; Oral tablet 10 mg; Granules 4mg/packet
Zafirlukast	Accolate®	10-20 mg once daily	Same as above	Tablets 10 mg, 20 mg

Inhaled Corticosteroids- Drugs for Nasal Allergies

Generic Name	Brand Name	Dose	Mechanism of Action	Dosage Form
Budesonide	Rhinocort® Aqua	1 spray each nostril once daily	Decreases the release of inflammatory factors.	Nasal Spray 32 mcg/spray 8.6 gm/inhaler, 120 sprays
Flunisolide	Nasarel®	2 sprays each nostril twice daily	Same as above	Nasarel 29 mcg/spray, 200 sprays/unit, 25 ml
Fluticasone	Flonase®	1 spray each nostril once daily	Same as above	Flonase® 50 mcg/spray, 16 gm/unit, 120 sprays/unit
Mometasone	Nasonex®	2 sprays each nostril once daily	Same as above	Nasonex® 50 mcg/spray, 17 gm/unit, 120 sprays/unit
Triamcinolone	Nasacort® AQ	2 sprays each nostril once daily	Same as above	Nasacort® AQ 55 mcg/spray, 16.5 grams/container, 120 sprays

Antihistamines - Sedating

Generic Name	Brand Name	Dose	Mechanism of Action	Dosage Form
Brompheniramine	Lodrane® 12 Hour, Lodrane® 24, Lodrane® XR	Lodrane® 12 Hour: 1-2 tablets every 12 hours as needed, max 4 tabs/24 hours	Blocks histamine receptor thus stopping nasal discharge.	Lodrane® 12 Hour
Chlorpheniramine	Chlor-trimeton®	1 tablet every 4 hours as needed	Same as above	Tablets 2 mg, 4 mg, 12 mg extended release tablets
Diphenhydramine	Benadryl®	1 tablet every 6 hours as needed	Same as above	Tablets 25 mg, Capsules 25 mg, Oral Solution 12.5 mg/5ml

Antihistamines - Non-Sedating

Generic Name	Brand Name	Dose	Mechanism of Action	Dosage Form
Cetirizine	Zyrtec®	1 tablet once daily	Same as above	Tablets 5 mg, 10 mg, Chewable tablet 5 mg, 10 mg, Syrup 5 mg/5ml
Fexofenadine	Allegra®	Adult 180 mg once daily	Same as above	Tablets 30 mg, 60 mg, 180 mg, Suspension 6 mg/ml
Loratadine	Claritin®	1 tablet once daily	Same as above	Tablet 10 mg, orally disintegrating tablet 10 mg, Syrup 1 mg/ml

Cystic Fibrosis				
Generic Name	Brand Name	Dose	Mechanism of Action	Dosage Form
Acetylcysteine	Mucomyst®	Inhale by nebulization 3-5 ml of 20% solution 3 to 4 times daily	Breaks mucus apart; its free sulfhydryl group breaks the disulfide bonds in mucus	Solution 10%, 20% available as 4 ml, 10 ml, 30 ml
Dornase Alfa	Pulmozyme®	2.5 mg once daily with selected nebulizers	Selectively cleaves the excess DNA strands, decreasing mucus viscosity, allowing the body to better remove it.	Solution for nebulization 1 mg/ml
Ivacaftor	Kalydeco®	A 150 mg tablet every 12 hours with fat containing food	Improves the function of a defective protein that causes cystic fibrosis.	Tablet 150 mg
Tobramycin	Tobi®	Inhale nebulized 80 mg twice daily	Antibiotic that kills infections associated with cystic fibrosis.	Solution for nebulization

Emphysema				
Generic Name	Brand Name	Dose	Mechanism of Action	Dosage Form
Alpha-1-Proteinase Inhibitor	Prolastin®	Inject IV 60 mg/kg once a week	Increases alpha-1-antitrypsin	IV

Page 134

CHAPTER 19

ESTROGENS AND TESTOSTERONE

Estrogen Agonists	Estrogen Antagonists		Progestins	Testosterone
Estradiol Conjugated Estrogens	**Selective Estrogen Receptor Modulators:** Raloxifene Tamoxifen Toremifene Clomiphene **Estrogen Receptor Antagonist:** Fulvestrant	**Aromatase Inhibitors:** Exemestane Anastrozole Letrozole **Decreased Estrogen Production:** Danazol	Medroxyprogesterone Megestrol Progesterone	**Agonists:** Fluoxymesterone Methyltestosterone Oxandrolone Testosterone **Antagonists:** Finasteride Dutasteride Flutamide

Estrogens have several clinical functions: 1) treating hypogonadism, 2) oral contraceptives, and 3) hormone replacement therapy. Selective estrogen receptor modulators have several purposes including: 1) treating hormone-responsive breast cancer, (tamoxifen) 2) preventing osteoporosis (raloxifene), and 3) stimulating ovulation (clomiphene).

Fulvestrant is an estrogen antagonist that treats breast cancer in patients who have tried tamoxifene and it did not work.

Testosterone supplements treat hypogonadism in adolescents. Recently, the use of testosterone supplements as replacement therapy has surged in middle aged men.

Estrogen, progesterone, and testosterone are hormones. Estrogen and testosterone cause the development and maintenance of secondary sex characteristics. Progesterone influences ovulation, menstruation, and pregnancy. Estrogen also influences ovulation. Breast tissue, endometrium, ovaries, and bone are sensitive to estrogen.

Multiple steps influence ovulation. Briefly using the hypothalamus as a starting point, it releases gonadotropin-releasing hormone (GnRH), which stimulates the anterior pituitary gland to release both follicle-stimulating hormone (FSH) and luteinizing hormone (LH). FSH and LH control the growth of a follicle (which turns into an ovum). The follicle and ovaries produce estrogen, which then causes the anterior pituitary to secrete more LH; ultimately, as a result of the combined actions of FSH, LH, and estrogen, ovulation occurs. Later, estrogen and progesterone cause negative feedback at the hypothalamus and anterior pituitary glands.

Separate from ovulation, LH and FSH both travel through the blood to the ovaries and testes, both of which then produce testosterone; ovaries then convert some of the testosterone to estrogen; ovaries also produce progesterone. Ovaries release some testosterone, into the blood, which, after arrival inside target cells (breast, endometrium, bone) is then transformed into estrogen by the enzyme aromatase. Estrogen then performs its normal biological functions in these tissues.

In males, at target cells, testosterone is transformed into the substantially more biologically active dihydrotestosterone by the enzyme 5-alpha-reductase. Testosterone then induces gene transcription, resulting in muscle growth and other biological responses. In males, blood levels of testosterone stay relatively constant from the onset of puberty through middle to old age.

ESTROGEN

Estradiol is the main estrogen; however estrone and estriol also circulate, but they have little biological activity relative to estrogen. Estradiol is indicated to treat: menopausal vasomotor symptoms; vulvar and vaginal atrophy resulting from menopause; hypoestrogenism; palliative treatment of certain breast cancers in women and metastatic cancer in men; advanced androgen-dependent carcinoma of the prostate; and prevention of osteoporosis in women.

Estrogens and progestins are used primarily for hormone replacement therapy (usually during menopause) and contraception. Various estrogens are used as contraceptives. Estrogens are always used in combination with a progestin for contraceptive purposes. Progestins can be used alone as contraceptives.

Estradiol is contraindicated in the following conditions: undiagnosed abnormal genital bleeding; breast cancer except for patients being treated for metastatic disease; known or suspected estrogen-dependent neoplasia; deep vein thrombosis or pulmonary embolism or history of these conditions; active or recent (within a year) arterial thromboembolic disease (stroke or myocardial infarction); liver dysfunction or disease; known or suspected pregnancy.

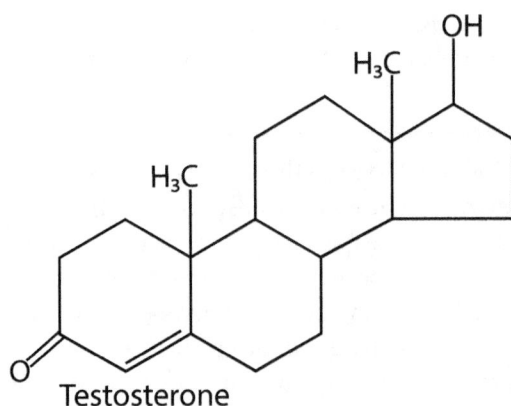

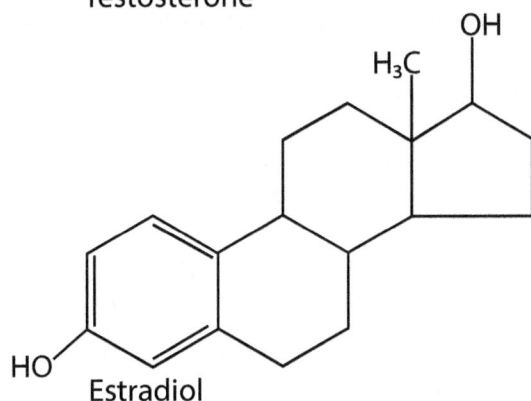

Testosterone

Estradiol

Estrogen Receptor Antagonist

Estrogen can promote cancer growth. Fulvestrant, an estrogen receptor antagonist, binds with estrogen receptors, preventing estrogen from binding with cancerous cells; thus slowing their growth. It treats hormone receptor positive metastatic breast cancer in post-menopausal women, after using anti-estrogen therapy. Doses should be administered over 1 to 2 minutes to reduce problems with bleeding. Patients may experience increased liver enzymes levels of ALT, AST, and ALP.

SELECTIVE ESTROGEN RECEPTOR MODULATORS

Selective estrogen receptor modulators (SERM) are neither pure antagonists nor pure agonists; rather they are a mixture of both. Clomiphene stimulates ovulation; thus allowing for the possibility of pregnancy. Clomiphene is a partial agonist in the ovaries and an antagonist in the pituitary gland and hypothalamus. As an antagonist of estrogen in the anterior pituitary gland and hypothalamus, it stops the negative feed-back loop of estrogen. Consequently, the hypothalamus releases gonadotropin-releasing hormone (GnRH). Several additional steps then occur. GnRH causes the anterior pituitary gland to release luteinizing hormone (LH) and follicle-stimulating hormone (FSH). FSH causes follicle growth. The follicle releases estrogens thus reinforcing its own growth; and finally the pituitary's release of LH causes ovulation.

Raloxifene is approved for the prevention of osteoporosis in post-menopausal women and the prevention of breast cancer. It is an agonist at estrogen receptors in bone, and it is an antagonist at receptors in breast tissue and in the endometrium. It is dosed once daily.

Tamoxifen is approved for the prevention of breast cancer in women who are at high risk of developing it. Tamoxifen is an antagonist of estrogen receptors in breast tissue; however, it is a partial agonist in endometrial tissue. Its partial agonist behavior in endometrial tissue may lead to the development of endometrial cancer; consequently, it should not be used for more than 5 years. Hypercalcemia has occurred in patients with breast cancer that has metastasized to bones. Tamoxifen should be discontinued if hypercalcemia cannot be controlled. Further, tamoxifen can cause deep vein thrombosis and pulmonary embolism.

Tamoxifen is also known to cause cataracts.

AROMATASE INHIBITORS

Anastrozole, letrozole, and exemestane prevent the enzyme aromatase from converting testosterone to estrogen. Each is approved for the treatment of breast cancer. These drugs are highly effective at preventing aromatase from converting testosterone to estrogen. They are so effective at reducing the production of estrogen that each has a warning stating that decreases in bone mineral density may occur. Patients should take steps to prevent osteoporosis while taking these drugs. Each of these causes hot flashes in about 20% of patients.

TESTOSTERONE

Testosterone treats hypogonadism, delayed puberty, and impotence. It can be used as a palliative treatment for metastatic breast cancer in females. Testosterone levels decrease as a male ages. Prescription testosterone is used to increase testosterone levels in older males, thus increasing muscle mass, increasing energy, and improving sex drive.

In the blood, testosterone binds to albumin and sex hormone-binding globulin (SHBG). When albumin or SHBG reach target cells, they release testosterone; it then diffuses through the cell membrane into the cytoplasm of the target cell. In the cytoplasm of the cell, the enzyme 5-alpha-reductase transforms testosterone to dihydrotestosterone. Dihydrotestosterone has substantially more biological activity relative to testosterone. In the cytoplasm, dihydrotestosterone binds with the androgen receptor; that complex of dihydrotestosterone and androgen receptor then diffuses into the nucleus of the cell. In the nucleus, that complex then binds with DNA, causing the transcription of genes that are dependent on androgens for activation.

5-Alpha-Reductase Inhibitors

Finasteride and dutasteride treat benign prostatic hyperplasia (BPH) to improve symptoms, reduce urinary retention, and reduce the need for surgery. Finasteride also treats hair loss in males. Both reduce prostate-specific antigen (PSA) levels by over 50%. Finasteride and dutasteride prevent 5-alpha-reductase from converting testosterone to dihydrotestosterone. Dihydrotestosterone binds with the cytoplasmic androgen receptor with a dramatically higher affinity than testosterone itself. By preventing the formation of dihydrotestosterone, mainly testosterone binds with the androgen receptor, which occurs at a much lower rate than dihydrotestosterone, slowing progression of BPH.

Impotence and decreased libido are the major common side-effects. Although the occurrence is minimal, both may increase the risk of high-grade prostate cancer; accordingly, patients should be closely monitored for any signs of prostate cancer. Finasteride may be used in combination with doxazosin for an even greater benefit than either alone. Dutasteride may be combined with tamsulosin for a synergistic effect. Both are administered once daily. Finasteride does not have any clinically significant drug interactions. Dutasteride's metabolism may be inhibited by strong CYP3A4 inhibitors.

Androgen Receptor Antagonists

Flutamide, an antagonist at testosterone receptors, treats prostate cancer. It is administered orally at 250 mg every 8 hours. Rarely, it causes hepatic failure. Consequently, it is contraindicated in patients with hepatic impairment. Spironolactone, in addition to being a diuretic, can be used as an antagonist at the androgen receptor; as an androgen receptor antagonist, it treats hirsutism (excess facial hair) in women.

Estrogens				
Generic Name	Brand Name	Use	Dose	Mechanism of Action
Conjugated Estrogens	Premarin®	Treats vasomotor symptoms caused by menopause	Initial dose 0.3 mg daily, increase if needed, use lowest possible dose	Replaces estrogen the body would normally produce, thus decreasing hot flashes and sweating
Estradiol	Climara®, Estrace®, Estring®, Femring®, Vagifem®, Vivelle®, Vivelle Dot®	Treats vasomotor symptoms caused by menopause, treats vulvar and vaginal atrophy	Adult oral dose is 0.5 mg -2 mg once daily	Replaces estrogen the body would normally produce, thus decreasing hot flashes and sweating

Selective Estrogen Receptor Modulators				
Clomiphene	Clomid®	Treats infertility in anovulatory women	50 mg orally once daily for 5 days, start on or about 5th day of cycle	Inhibits normal estrogen negative feed-back, thus allowing ovulation
Raloxifene	Evista®	Treats and prevents osteoporosis in post-menopause Risk reduction for invasive breast cancer	Osteoporosis or risk reduction for invasive breast cancer: 60 mg once daily	Antagonist at breast estrogen receptors; agonist at estrogen receptors in bone
Tamoxifen	Nolvadex®	Adjuvant treatment of breast cancer, metastatic breast cancer, axillary node-negative breast cancer in women, ductal carcinoma in situ	Prevention of breast cancer, oral dose: 10 mg twice daily for 5 years	Antagonist at breast estrogen receptors
Toremifene	Fareston®	Treats post-menopausal metastatic breast cancer	60 mg orally once daily	Same as above

Anti-Estrogens : Complete Antagonists at All Receptors				
Generic Name	Brand Name	Clinical Use	Dose	Mechanism of Action
Fulvestrant	Faslodex®	Treats hormone receptor positive metastatic breast cancer, in patients who have tried tamoxifen but it did not work	IM dose: 250 mg once every 30 days	As an antagonist, it binds with estrogen receptors, thus preventing gene expression

Anti-Estrogens: Aromatase Inhibitors

Generic Name	Brand Name	Clinical Use	Dose	Mechanism of Action
Anastrozole	Arimidex®	Treats locally advanced and metastatic breast cancer	1 mg orally once daily	Reversibly blocks aromatase
Exemestane	Aromasin®	Treats advanced breast cancer	25 mg orally once daily	Exemestane irreversibly blocks the active site of aromatase
Letrozole	Femara®	Treats locally advanced and metastatic breast cancer	2.5 mg orally once daily	Reversibly blocks aromatase

Testosterone

Generic Name	Brand Name	Clinical Use	Dose	Mechanism of Action
Fluoxymesterone	Halotestin	Replaces testosterone in males who are deficient, palliative treatment of breast cancer	Hypogonadism, oral dose: 5-20 mg a day; Inoperable breast cancer: 10-40 mg a daily for 1 to 3 months	Functions as normal testosterone does
Methyltestosterone	Android® Testred®	Hypogonadism, delayed puberty, impotence, palliative treatment of metastatic breast cancer	Hypogonadism, oral dose: 10-40 mg once a day; breast cancer, oral dose: 50-200 mg/day	Same as above
Oxandrolone	Oxandrin®	Promotes weight gain after weight loss following surgery, chronic infections, or severe trauma	Adult doses vary, 2.5 mg to 20 mg total daily dose in 2 to 4 divided doses. Therapy should last for 2 to 4 weeks and can be repeated intermittently	Same as above
Testosterone cypionate	Depo-Testosterone®	Replaces testosterone for hypogonadism	50 mg to 400 mg intramuscularly every 2 to 4 weeks	Same as above

Testosterone Antagonists

Generic Name	Brand Name	Clinical Use	Dose	Mechanism of Action
Dutasteride	Avodart®	Benign prostatic hyperplasia	0.5 mg once daily	Prevent 5-alpha-reductase from converting testosterone to dihydrotestosterone
Finasteride	Proscar®	Benign prostatic hyperplasia	5 mg once daily	Same as above
Flutamide	Eulexin	Metastatic carcinoma of the prostate	250 mg 3 times daily at 8 hour intervals	Antagonist at testosterone receptors

CHAPTER 20

ANTI-DIABETIC DRUGS

Rapid-Acting Insulin	Insulin Short-Acting	Intermediate Acting Insulin	Long-Acting Insulin	Combination Insulins
Insulin Aspart Insulin Glulisine Insulin Lispro	Insulin Regular	Insulin NPH (isophane suspension)	Insulin Detemir Insulin Glargine	Insulin Aspart protamine suspension and insulin aspart; Insulin Lispro protamine and insulin lispro; Insulin NPH suspension and insulin regular

Oral Diabetic Drugs

Biguanide	Alpha-glucosidase Inhibitors	Dipeptidyl Peptidase Inhibitors	Meglitinides	Sulfonylureas	Thiazolidinediones
Metformin	Acarbose Miglitol	Linagliptin Saxagliptin Sitagliptin	Nateglinide Repaglinide	First Generation: Chlorpropamide Tolazamide Tolbutamide Second Generation: Glimepiride Glipizide Glyburide	Pioglitazone Rosiglitazone

Type 1 diabetes usually begins during childhood. Type 1 diabetes, characterized by the pancreas not producing any insulin at all, requires patients to inject insulin. Type 2 diabetes, commonly called adult onset diabetes, is characterized by the body's inability to use the insulin that the pancreas does produce. All insulin products have the same mechanism of action as endogenous insulin; they differ in their onset of action and duration of action. Altering insulin's amino acid sequence, alters its onset of action and duration of action. Also, altering the suspension that it is in, also alters its duration of action.

Oral anti-diabetic drugs have different mechanisms of action. Metformin and thiazolidinediones increases cells' sensitivity to insulin, allowing for greater uptake of glucose into cells. Alpha-glucosidase inhibitors prevent the metabolism of carbohydrates to glucose; thus preventing blood sugar levels from rising after meals. Dipeptidyl peptidase inhibitors keep levels of gastric inhibitory peptide elevated after meals; gastric inhibitory peptide stimulates insulin release; dipeptidyl peptidase metabolizes gastric inhibitory peptide. Meglitinides and sulfonylureas stimulate pancreatic beta cells to secrete insulin.

Page 142

The cause(s) of type I diabetes is unknown; physicians treat type I diabetes with insulin injections. Type II diabetes results from an inability to effectively transfer glucose from the blood stream into cells where it can be used. Physicians have several choices for treating Type II diabetes; treatment plans vary according to the severity of the symptoms and individual characteristics of the patient. Usually physicians start patients on oral medications first and then decide whether to add insulin based on the patient's response. Physicians can pick from alpha-glucosidase inhibitors, biguanides, dipeptidyl peptidase IV inhibitors (DPP-IV), meglitinides, sulfonylureas, and thiazolidinediones.

Pancreatic beta cells produce insulin. The pancreas releases insulin into the blood stream; insulin allows all cells to use glucose for energy. Insulin's action are particularly important at adipose cells, liver cells, and muscle cells because these cells are the main cells that either use glucose or store it as energy. In adipose cells, insulin causes glucose and fatty acids to be combined into triglycerides, which is one way the body stores energy. In muscle cells, insulin causes cells to produce glycogen, which is produced from many individual units of glucose. Insulin causes liver cells to produce glycogen and triglycerides.

In contrast, glucagon, an energy releasing hormone, raises blood sugar when it is too low. Pancreatic alpha-cells produce glucagon. Glucagon reverses what insulin does. It causes hepatic glycogenolysis (the conversion of glycogen to glucose) and gluconeogenesis (the production of glucose separate from the breakdown of glycogen). Glucagon is available as a commercially produced drug. Patients with type I diabetes should keep a glucagon injection on-hand for emergencies.

DRUGS

INSULIN

Insulin products are usually categorized according to their duration of action. Today, rapid-acting, short-acting, intermediate-acting, intermediate to long-acting, long-acting, and combination products are available. Combination products combine a short-acting insulin with a longer acting insulin to produce a product that acts quickly and lasts for a long-time. Today, all insulin is human insulin.

Insulin is made of two chains of amino acids, an "A" chain and a "B" chain. The A chain has 30 amino acids and the B chain has 21 amino acids. The A chain and the B chain are linked to each other by two disulfide bonds. The first disulfide bond is between cysteine A7 and cysteine B7; the second disulfide bond is between cysteine A20 and cysteine B19.

Altering one or more amino acid residues, produces insulin analogs. Three short acting insulin analogs are insulin aspart, insulin glulisine, and insulin lispro. Insulin aspart is formed by changing proline at B28 to aspartic acid. Insulin glulisine is formed by changing aspartic acid at B3 to lysine and also changing lysine at B29 to glutamic acid. Insulin lispro is formed by changing proline at B28 to lysine and lysine at B29 to proline. Two long acting insulins are insulin detemir and insulin glargine. Insulin detemir is formed by adding myristoyl (a saturated fatty acid) to the B29 lysine residue. Insulin glargine is formed by adding two arginine amino acids to the end of the B chain (making it a total of 32 amino acid residues) and changing asparagine A21 to glycine; this analog is less soluble at physiologic pH (7.4), and, consequently, it absorbs more slowly, translating into a delayed onset of action, but prolonged half-life.

Another long-acting insulin is insulin neutral protamine hagedorn (insulin NPH, insulin isophane). Rather than alter the amino acid sequence of insulin, the developers mixed insulin, zinc, and protamine into a solution of phosphate buffer, creating a long-acting suspension of insulin. The zinc and protamine give it a cloudy appearance, in contrast to other single product insulins.

INSULIN DOSING

Of course, insulin doses vary considerably from patient to patient. Insulin is usually initially dosed at 0.5-1 units/kg/day administered as divided doses. Some patients adjust their dose based on the amount of carbohydrates they consume and/or based on their current blood sugar level. Due to the risk of hypoglycemia, some physicians start patients on lower doses. Outside of a medical emergency, doses should be started low and slowly increased as necessary.

Patients have considerable choices in deciding which insulins to use. The faster acting and long acting insulins are quite expensive. If necessary, a patient can use just regular insulin and insulin NPH, which are much less expensive. Longer-acting insulins may provide better blood sugar control for most patients, but can drop blood sugar too low in some patients.

Exenatide, known as an incretin mimetic, in an injection used to treat type II diabetes. It stimulates pancreatic beta cells to release insulin and decreases abnormally high levels of glucagon (glucagon increases blood sugar levels). It also delays gastric emptying which decreases the rate at which sugars enter the blood stream. Exenatide is for subcutaneous administration only. It is injected within 60 minutes of the two main meals of the day, at least two hours apart. For the first month, patients should receive 5 mcg twice daily, then increased to 10 mcg twice daily. It may cause pancreatitis, which necessitates withdrawal of the medication.

There have been reports of renal impairment.

ORAL MEDICATIONS FOR DIABETES

Oral anti-hyperglycemic medications include alpha-glucosidase inhibitors, biguanide, dipeptidyl peptidase inhibitors, meglitinides, sulfonylureas (first and second generations), and thiazolidinediones. Oral medications treat type 2 diabetes.

ALPHA-GLUCOSIDASE INHIBITORS

Acarbose and miglitol inhibit the enzyme alpha-glucosidase from converting carbohydrates (chains of sugar molecules) to glucose; ultimately they decrease blood glucose levels after meals (postprandial). They can be used as mono-therapy with dietary restrictions or they can be used with a sulfonylurea, if dietary restrictions alone are insufficient to control blood sugar levels. They are approved to treat type II diabetes. They are not metabolized and they do not inhibit or induce any CYP isoenzymes.

BIGUANIDE

Metformin, presently the only available biguanide, is the drug of choice for treating type II diabetes. It increases cells' sensitivity to insulin, allowing for greater uptake of glucose into cells. Unless contraindicated, clinicians usually start patients with type II diabetes on metformin, and, then, if necessary, add a second medication. Metformin is contraindicated with renal disease or renal dysfunction, acute myocardial infarction, septicemia, metabolic acidosis, or diabetic keto-acidosis. Metformin has a black box warning for lactic acidosis. Metformin should be discontinued

prior to the administration of iodinated contrast media because of the risk of a decrease in renal function. Further, it commonly causes gastrointestinal disturbances. All patients should stay well hydrated to decrease the risk of side-effects, especially lactic acidosis.

DIPEPTIDYL PEPTIDASE INHIBITORS

Glucose-dependent insulinotropic polypeptide, also known as gastric inhibitory peptide (GIP), stimulates insulin secretion, thus lowering blood sugar levels. Dipeptidyl peptidase (DPP) is an enzyme that inactivates GIP; thus the enzyme DPP can keep blood sugar levels high by preventing GIP from stimulating insulin secretion. Inhibiting DPP allows GIP to lower blood sugar. Linagliptin, saxagliptin, and sitagliptin inhibit DPP, thus allowing GIP to lower blood sugar by stimulating insulin release. As a class, these drugs have limited side-effects and are generally well tolerated. They can be used with any of the following: insulin, metformin, sulfonylureas, or thiazolidinediones. They are approved to treat type II diabetes.

MEGLITINIDES

Nateglinide and repaglinide stimulate pancreatic beta cells to secrete insulin. They block potassium channels, which causes calcium ions to enter beta cells, which causes beta cells to release insulin. They are approved to treat type II diabetes as monotherapy with diet restrictions and exercise. They can also be used with metformin or thiazolidinediones. Repaglinide is metabolized by CYP2C8 and CYP3A4. Strong inducers of either CYP2C8 or CYP3A4 lower blood levels of repaglinide; and strong inhibitors of either increase blood levels. Nateglinide is metabolized by CYP2C9 and CYP3A4; inhibitors of either increase blood levels of nateglinide; and inducers of either decrease blood levels of nateglinide. These drugs should be used cautiously in patients with hepatic impairment or severe renal dysfunction. Further, caution should be used in the elderly because of the risk of hypoglycemia.

SULFONYLUREAS

Sulfonylureas are divided into first generation and second generation drugs. All sulfonylureas stimulate beta cells to release insulin, reducing blood glucose levels. Specifically, sulfonylureas inhibit certain potassium channels (those dependent on ATP) of beta cells ultimately causing beta cells to release insulin. They may also increase the sensitivity of cells to insulin and may decrease the liver's release of glucose into the bloodstream.

Second generation sulfonylureas are used as monotherapy (to treat type II diabetes) with diet restrictions and exercise; they are also used with metformin. First generation sulfonylureas commonly cause hypoglycemia. The risk of severe hypoglycemia limits use of first generation sulfonylureas. Second generation sulfonylureas can still cause hypoglycemia, but not as often as first generation drugs.

Alcohol, when combined with a sulfonylurea, can cause hypoglycemia. Other drugs that, when combined with a sulfonylurea, can cause hypoglycemia include: warfarin, ketoconazole, fluconazole, sulfonamides, and tricyclic antidepressants. Drugs that can decrease the effectiveness of sulfonylureas include cholestyramine, phenytoin, rifampin, and thiazide diuretics.

Increased cellular glucose uptake, resulting from sulfonylurea use, may cause weight gain.

Hepatic impairment or renal insufficiency are contraindications for first generation sulfonylureas. Both generations are contraindicated for pregnant patients and mother's nursing. Both generations can increase or decrease the effects of numerous other drugs.

THIAZOLIDINEDIONES

Thiazolidinediones increase cells' sensitivity to insulin. Pioglitazone and rosiglitazone are agonists at the peroxisome-proliferation-activating receptor gamma (PPAR gamma). When the PPAR gamma nuclear receptor is stimulated by agonists, the receptor causes genes to produce proteins that increase a cell's sensitivity to insulin; thus the cell is able to draw glucose out of the bloodstream, effectively lowering blood sugar levels. Rosiglitazone is approved to treat type II diabetes as monotherapy with diet restrictions and exercise; or in combination with either a sulfonylurea or metformin; or in combination with both a sulfonylurea and metformin.

Pioglitazone is approved to treat type II diabetes as monotherapy with diet restrictions and exercise; or in combination with a sulfonylurea, metformin, or insulin. In contrast to other drugs used to treat diabetes, these two may take four to twelve weeks before blood sugar levels drop. Both of these drugs have black box warnings for possibly causing or exacerbating heart failure. Both are contraindicated in patients with NYHA Class III/IV heart failure. Further, both of these drugs can cause weight gain. Finally, women may be at increased risk of bone fracture as a result of using these drugs.

Insulin Rapid-Acting				
Generic Name	Brand Name	Onset	Duration in Hours	Peak Effect on Blood Sugar (hours)
Insulin Aspart	Novolog®	10 to 20 minutes	3 - 5	1 - 3
Insulin Glulisine	Apidra®	15 to 20 minutes	3 - 4	1 - 2
Insulin Lispro	Humalog®	15 to 30 minutes	3 - 5	0.5 - 2.5
Insulin Short-Acting				
Insulin Regular	Humulin® R Novolin® R	30 minutes to 1 hour	4 - 12	2.5 - 5
Insulin Intermediate-Acting				
Insulin NPH (isophane suspension)	Humulin® N Novolin® N	1 - 2 hours	14 - 24	4 - 12

Insulin - Long-Acting				
Insulin Detemir	Levemir®	3 - 4 hours	6 - 23	3 - 9
Insulin Glargine	Lantus®	3 - 4 hours	10 - 24	No peak
Combination Insulins				
Insulin Aspart protamine suspension and insulin aspart	Novolog® Mix 70/30	10 to 30 minutes	18 - 24	1 - 4
Insulin Lispro protamine and insulin lispro	Humalog® Mix 75/25	15 to 30 minutes	14 - 24	1 - 6.5
Insulin NPH suspension and insulin regular	Novolin® 70/30	30 minutes	18 - 24	2 - 12

Oral Medications to Lower Blood Sugar				
Generic Name	Brand Name	Dose	Dosage Form	Mechanism of Action
Alpha-glucosidase Inhibitors				
Acarbose	Precose®	25-50 mg 3 times daily	Tablets 25, 50, 100 mg	Inhibits the conversion of sucrose to glucose and fructose
Miglitol	Glyset®	25-100 mg 3 times daily	Tablets 25, 50, 100 mg	Same as above
Biguanides				
Metformin	Glucophage®, Glucophage® XR, Fortamet®, Glumetza®, Riomet®	500-2550 mg/day in divided doses	Glucophage® tablets 500, 850 mg; Glucophage® XR 500, 750 mg, Riomet® Solution 100 mg/ml	Improves cells' sensitivity to insulin, thus promoting the passage of glucose into cells
Dipeptidyl Peptidase IV Inhibitors				
Linagliptin	Tradjenta®	5mg once daily	Tablets 5 mg	Prolongs incretin levels, ultimately causing beta cells to produce more insulin and causes the pancreas to release that insulin
Saxagliptin	Onglyza®	Adult 2.5-5 mg once daily	Tablets 2.5 mg, 5 mg	Same as above
Sitagliptin	Januvia®	Adults 25-100 mg once daily	Tablet 25 mg, 50 mg, 100 mg	Same as above

Oral Medications to Lower Blood Sugar				
Generic Name	Brand Name	Dose	Dosage Form	Mechanism of Action
Meglitinides				

Page 146

Oral Medications to Lower Blood Sugar				
Generic Name	Brand Name	Dose	Dosage Form	Mechanism of Action
Nateglinide	Starlix®	Adult 60-120 mg 3 times daily	Tablets 60 mg, 120 mg	Stimulates beta cells to release insulin
Repaglinide	Prandin®	Adult 0.5-4 mg with meals, max dose of 16 mg/day	Tablets 0.5, 1, 2 mg	Same as above
Sulfonylureas First Generation				
Chlorpropamide	Diabinese®	Adult 100-250 mg once daily	Tablets 100, 250 mg	Stimulates beta cells to release insulin
Tolazamide	Tolinase	Adult 250-1000 mg daily	Tablets 250, 500 mg	Same as above
Tolbutamide	Orinase®	Adult 250-2000 mg/day as one dose or divided doses	Tablet 500 mg	Same as above
Sulfonylureas Second Generation				
Generic	Brand	Dose	Dosage Form	Mechanism of Action
Glimepiride	Amaryl®	Adult dose 1 mg-4 mg once daily	Tablets 1, 2, 4 mg	Stimulates beta cells to release insulin, causes the liver to decrease glucose production, increases insulin sensitivity at cells
Glipizide	Glucotrol®, Glucotrol® Xl	Adult dose 5 mg-10 mg once daily, max dose of 20 mg daily	Tablets 5 mg, 10 mg; Extended release: 2.5 mg, 5 mg, 10 mg	Same as above
Glyburide	Diabeta®, Micronase®, Glynase® PresTab	Adult dose 1.25 mg - 20 mg daily in single or divided doses. Dose cautiously in elderly	Diabeta® tablets: 1.25 mg, 2.5 mg, 5 mg; Glynase® PresTab: 1.5 mg, 3 mg, 6 mg	Same as above
Thiazolidinediones				
Pioglitazone	Actos®	Adult dose 15 mg -45 mg once daily	Tablets 15 mg, 30 mg, 45 mg	Increases cells' sensitivity to insulin
Rosiglitazone	Avandia ®(special availability)	Adult dose 2 mg-8 mg once daily	Tablets 2 mg, 4 mg, 8 mg	Same as above

CHAPTER 21

THYROID DRUGS

Hypothyroidism	Hyperthyroidism
Replace levothyroxine	Limit levothyroxine production
Levothyroxine Liothyronine Liotrix Thyroid Desiccated	Potassium Iodide and Iodine Methimazole Propylthiouracil

Hypothyroidism occurs more commonly than hyperthyroidism. Levothyroxine is the most commonly used drug to treat hypothyroidism. It is available in many different strengths, reflecting the highly individualized doses required to adequately treat patients. TSH levels must be checked before starting therapy and three months after starting therapy to check for effectiveness. Calcium and iron salts bind with levothyroxine in the GI tract, diminishing levothyroxine's absorption. Hyperthyroidism is treated by decreasing the production of levothyroxine. Thyroid storm, resulting from overdoses of levothyroxine or autoimmune disease, is a medical emergency requiring immediate treatment, usually with propylthiouracil or methimazole, along with other medications and medical interventions.

The thyroid gland produces thyroxine (T4) and tri-iodothyronine (T3) (T4 is not believed to be biologically active). T3 controls the body's energy use and normal growth and development. It influences all metabolic processes. In essence, the thyroid controls how fast or slow the body works as a whole. Too much T3 causes weight loss, excess energy, weakness, heat intolerance, sweating, fast heart-rate, and goiter. In contrast, too little T3 may cause cold intolerance, (T3 causes heat production as a byproduct of metabolism) weight gain, fatigue, hoarseness, constipation, slow heart-rate, goiter, and anemia, among other health problems.

Normally, the hypothalamus and anterior pituitary gland jointly regulate the thyroid's production of T4 and T3. A negative feed-back loop regulates the thyroid's production of T3 and T4. Starting with the hypothalamus, it releases thyrotropin-releasing hormone (TRH). TRH stimulates the anterior pituitary gland to release thyroid-stimulating hormone (TSH). TSH, in turn, causes the thyroid gland to produce and release T3 and T4 into the blood. As the negative feed-back, T4 and T3 cause the hypothalamus to release less TRH, causing the anterior pituitary gland to release less TSH. Hashimoto's thyroiditis or Grave's disease can cause this negative feed-back loop to malfunction.

HYPOTHYROIDISM

Hypothyroidism results from a shortage of T-3. Hashimoto's Disease or other unknown causes may be the source of hypothyroidism. In Hashimoto's disease, an auto-antibody destroys the thyroid gland itself, preventing the thyroid gland from producing and releasing T4 and T3. Consequently, T4 and T3 are incapable of providing the normal negative feed-back to the hypothalamus and pituitary gland, resulting in increased levels of TRH and TSH. Levothyroxine and related products treat hypothyroidism.

HYPERTHYROIDISM

Hyperthyroidism results from an excess of T3. Grave's disease or other unknown causes may be the source of hyperthyroidism. Grave's disease results from an auto-antibody stimulating the thyroid gland to produce excess T4 and T3, then releasing them into the blood stream. Once in the blood stream, T3 and T4 eventually circulate to the hypothalamus and anterior pituitary gland, suppressing the release of TRH and TSH, resulting in low blood levels of TSH and TRH. Methimazole and propylthiouracil treat Grave's disease by preventing T3 and T4 production. Hyperthyroidism can be treated with potassium iodide and iodine (2 ingredients together in one compound), methimazole, and propylthiouracil. If drug treatment is unsuccessful, then surgery may be necessary to remove the gland.

DRUGS

LEVOTHYROXINE

Levothyroxine, a synthetic version of T-4, which is converted by the body to the biologically active T3, treats hypothyroidism. Liothyronine, a synthetic T-3, also treats hypothyroidism. Some patients simultaneously use both levothyroxine and liothyronine. Also, T-3 and T-4 are available in one tablet. In general, most patients do well with levothyroxine as monotherapy. Levothyroxine also treats hypothyroidism in newborns. Hypothyroidism in newborns prevents normal brain development, resulting in severe neurological deficits.

Levothyroxine (T4) has a half-life of 6 days; T3 has a half-life of about 1 day; this makes levothyroxine preferable to other drugs because blood levels stay more stable. T4 is more highly bound to plasma proteins than T3, which explains its longer half-life.

The general initial dose of levothyroxine is 1.7 mcg/kg/day. Levothyroxine should be taken at least 30 minutes before breakfast. A TSH level is usually drawn around two to three months, and then clinicians decide whether to change the dose. As with most drugs, start low, and go slow until an appropriate dose is found.

Many drugs decrease absorption of levothyroxine, including aluminum and/or magnesium antacids, simethicone, cholestyramine, colestipol, calcium carbonate, kayexalate, ferrous sulfate, orlistat, and sucralfate. Carbamazepine, phenytoin, phenobarbital, and rifampin induce hepatic metabolism of levothyroxine, thus lowering its levels. Levothyroxine stimulates the break down of vitamin K-dependent clotting factors; this can potentiate warfarin's activity, leading to increased bleeding. Amiodarone can interfere with the thyroid gland and thyroid treatment in patients with a functioning thyroid gland. Amiodarone tablets contain iodide, which may ultimately cause hypothyroidism or hyperthyroidism

Excessive doses of thyroid hormone replacement drugs may cause thyrotoxicosis, necessitating emergency medical treatment.

METHIMAZOLE

Methimazole treats hyperthyroidism. It may be used long-term or short-term until surgery can be performed. It stops the thyroid gland from attaching iodine to tyrosyl, thus ultimately preventing the production of T3 and T4.

Methimazole may cause agranulocytosis. Patients' bone marrow function should be monitored. Further, methimazole may cause severe hepatic problems, even causing death; monitor patients closely. Methimazole can cause fetal harm, and it should be avoided in pregnant patients. Methimazole should not be used by nursing mothers because it is excreted in breast milk; as noted above, hypothyroidism in infants can cause developmental problems.

Methimazole may increase the affects of warfarin; monitor patients' INRs closely. Hyperthyroidism may require higher doses of several medications. Beta blockers, digoxin, and theophylline may all require lower doses once a patient's hyperthyroidism is controlled by methimazole.

PROPYLTHIOURACIL

Propylthiouracil has the same mechanism of action as methimazole. Propylthiouracil treats patients with Grave's Disease hyperthyroidism or multinodular goiter in patients who cannot use methimazole, and radioactive iodine treatment and surgery are not appropriate therapy. Propylthiouracil is a last choice to treat hyperthyroidism. Propylthiouracil can cause severe liver injury and acute liver failure (sometimes fatal). Sometimes liver transplantation has been required.

Propylthiouracil may increase the affects of warfarin, increasing a patient's INR; close monitoring of a patient's INR is warranted when these medications are used together. When a patient's hyperthyroidism is controlled, doses of digitalis (digoxin), beta-blockers, and/or theophylline may need to lowered.

Hypothyroid Medications

Generic Name	Brand Name	Dose	Dosage Form	Mechanism of Action
Levothyroxine	Synthroid® Levoxyl® Levothroid®	Adult 25-300 mcg once daily	Tablets 25, 50, 75, 88, 100, 112, 125, 137, 150, 175, 200, 300 mcg; Injection: 100 mcg/vial, 500 mcg/vial	Replaces T4
Liothyronine	Cytomel®, Triostat®	Adult 5-50 mcg once daily	Tablets 5, 25, 50 mcg; Triostat® injection 10 mcg/ml (1ml)	Replaces T3
Liotrix	Thyrolar®	Adult: 1/4 - 3 grains once daily	Tablets 1/4, 1/2, 1, 2, 3 grains	Replaces T3 and T4
Thyroid Desiccated	Armour® Thyroid	Adult 15-300 mg once daily	Tablets 15, 30, 60, 90, 120, 180, 240, 300 mg	Replaces T3 and T4

Hyperthyroid Medications

Generic Name	Brand Name	Dose	Dosage Form	Mechanism of Action
Methimazole	Tapazole®	Initial adult dose for mild hyperthyroidism 5 mg three times daily	Tablets 5 mg, 10 mg	Stops the thyroid gland from attaching iodine to tyrosyl, thus ultimately preventing the production of T3 and T4
Potassium Iodide and Iodine	Potassium Iodide and Iodine	Adult hyperthyroidism 4-8 drops every 6-8 hours, start at least one hour after propylthiouracil or methimazole	Solution: 100 mg/ml of Iodide and 50 mg/ml of Iodine	Temporarily inhibits synthesis of thyroid hormone, thus decreasing levels of T3 and T4; also prevents uptake of radioactive iodine into the thyroid gland, thus preventing thyroid cancer
Propylthiouracil	Propylthiouracil	Initial adult dose 100 mg 3 times daily, uncommonly 600 mg to 900 mg daily. Maintenance dose: 100 mg - 150 mg daily	Tablet 50 mg	Same as above

CHAPTER 22

ANTIBIOTICS

Cell Wall Inhibitors	Inhibitors of Protein Synthesis	Inhibitors of DNA Replication	Inhibitors of RNA Synthesis	Anti-Metabolites
Inhibitors of peptide cross-linking: Penicillins Cephalosporins **Enolpyruvyl Transferase Inhibitor (Blocking peptidoglycan synthesis):** Fosfomycin **Blocking peptidoglycan polymerization:** Vancomycin and Telavancin	**Inhibitors of the 30S Ribosomal Subunit:** Aminoglycosides Tetracycline Tetracycline derivatives **Inhibitors of the 50S Ribosomal Subunit:** Chloramphenicol Macrolides Lincosamides Streptogramins Oxazolidinone	**Topoisomerase Inhibitors:** Quinolones Fluoroquinolones	Rifabutin Rifampin	Sulfamethoxazole Sulfadiazine Trimethoprim

Cell wall inhibitors prevent construction of a functioning cell wall; this eventually leads to cell death. Protein synthesis inhibitors prevent bacteria from forming functional proteins necessary for life. Inhibitors of DNA replication prevent topoisomerase from unwinding DNA during DNA replication (unwinding of DNA is a critical step in DNA replication). Inhibitors of RNA synthesis prevent the formation of functional RNA. RNA is the messenger that is sent to the ribosomes to be decoded allowing protein synthesis.

Anti-metabolites prevent the formation of DNA base pairs. DNA is made of four different base pairs, which encode genetic information. Without these base pairs, DNA cannot be produced.

Antibiotics cause side-effects by affecting the good bacteria normally living in the gastrointestinal tract. Sometimes this requires treatment with other antibiotics.

Most bacteria are divided into three classes, gram positive, gram negative, and mycobacteria. Gram positive bacteria have thick cell walls made of peptidoglycan chains. These chains are made of amino acids and sugars. Peptidoglycan retains a purple dye when coated with the dye. Bacteria that retain the dye are called gram positive. In contrast, gram negative bacteria do not retain the dye because they have much less peptidoglycan in their cell walls, but have a layer of lipopolysaccharide located outside the peptidoglycan layer. Lipopolysaccharide does not retain the purple dye. Mycobacteria also have a lipid layer outside of the peptidoglycan layer, but this layer has different building blocks than gram-negative bacteria; these building blocks also protect bacteria.

Bacteria are also divided into aerobic, and anaerobic bacteria. Aerobic bacteria need oxygen to live. Anaerobic bacteria exist in one of three separate classes: 1) obligate anerobes die in the presence of oxygen; 2) aerotolerant bacteria can grow with or without oxygen; and 3) faculatative bacteria can live without oxygen by changing their means of producing energy without oxygen.

CELL WALL INHIBITORS

Bacterial cell wall synthesis follows three main steps: 1) murein monomer synthesis (building blocks of the wall) (murein and peptidoglycan are the same), 2) polymerization of murein monomers to form glycan chains, and 3) cross linking of the peptides located on glycan chains to complete the wall. Specific inhibitors exist for each of these three steps.

ENOLPYRUVYL TRANSFERASE INHIBITOR

Fosfomycin (bactericidal) inhibits peptidoglycan (murein) synthesis. Murein monomers are the individual building blocks of peptidoglycan chains. Fosfomycin blocks the active site of the enzyme enolpyruvate transferase from producing murein monomers. More specifically it prevents the joining of uridine diphosphate-N-acetylglucosamine and p-enolpyruvate. Fosfomycin is effective against E. coli, Klebsiella, and Serratia (all gram negative); all commonly involved in urinary tract infections. Fosfomycin has the advantage of having to be dosed (3 grams) only once, but it is considerably more expensive than older medications. Antacids reduce the absorption of fosfomycin.

Bacitracin, another inhibitor of murein monomer synthesis, works by blocking the enzyme dephosphorylase from dephosphorylating bactoprenyl diphosphate, thus stopping murein monomer synthesis. Bacitracin is used for skin or opthalmic infections. It can be used orally for *clostridium difficile* and vancomycin-resistant enterococci.

STOPPING PEPTIDOGLYCAN POLYMERIZATION

Vancomycin (bactericidal) and telavancin both inhibit the polymerization of peptidoglycan. Both bind to the bacterial cell wall, blocking peptidoglycan polymerization. Telavancin treats complicated skin and skin structure infections caused by susceptible gram-positive bacteria, including *staphylococcus aureus* (including methicllin susceptible and resistant isolates), *streptococcus pyogenes*, *streptococcus agalactiae*, *streptococcus anginosus* group, or *enterococcus*. Vancomycin treats methicillin-resistant staphylococcus aureus. Vancomycin causes red-man syndrome. Bacterial resistance to vancomycin is widespread.

INHIBITORS OF PEPTIDE CROSS-LINKING

All beta-lactam drugs inhibit the cross-linking of peptidoglycan chains by binding with transpeptidases (also known as "penicillin binding proteins" PBPs). Transpeptidases link one peptidoglycan chain with another chain. In particular, the beta-lactam ring binds with transpeptidase, preventing transpeptidase from working. Beta-Lactam drugs are divided into four main categories: penicillins (including amoxicillin and its derivatives), cephalosporins, carbapenems, and monobactams. The need for multiple drug classes derives from the fact that bacteria naturally develop resistance to antibiotics. Each class has a different structural ring next to the beta-lactam ring. The structural ring next to the beta-lactam ring prevents bacteria from inactivating the beta-lactam ring.

Each of these drugs causes the enzyme transpeptidase to bind with the carbonyl carbon (the carbon atom that is double-bonded to oxygen); after binding to one of these drugs, transpeptidase is unable to disconnect itself from the drug and consequently can no longer attach one chain of peptidoglycan to another chain of peptidoglycan. An individual peptidoglycan has two main parts: an amino-sugar part and peptide part that connects or bridges the amino-sugar-chain to a second amino-sugar-chain. The amino-sugar parts form

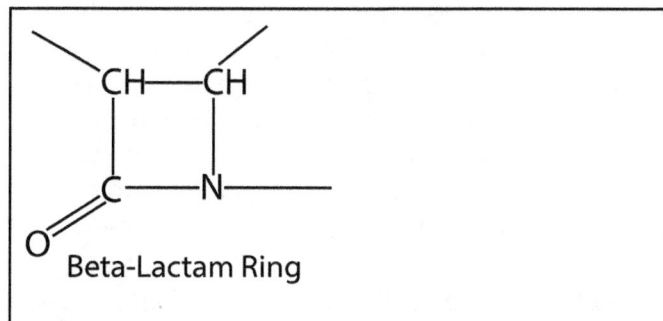

Beta-Lactam Ring

individual chains that normally completely encircle the bacteria. The peptide parts of each peptidoglycan connect the amino-sugar parts together to complete the wall.

PENICILLINS

The penicillin class is traditionally divided into four additional subclasses: 1) natural penicillins 2) penicillinase-resistant penicillins 3) broad spectrum aminopenicillins, and 4) extended spectrum penicillins anti-pseudomonas. Sometimes different names are used to describe these classes. Because of the structural differences between the classes, they have different spectrums of action against bacteria.

Group I includes penicillin G and penicillin V. Penicillin V is used to treat infections caused by penicillin sensitive *S. Aureus*. Penicillin G treats gram-positive bacteria including *streptococcus pyogenes* and *streptococcus pneumoniae*.

Group II includes cloxacillin, dicloxacillin, methicillin, nafcillin, and oxacillin. Group II penicillins are effective against staphylococcal infections. Their chemical structures make them more resistant to beta-lactamase. Beta-lactamase inactivates beta-lactam drugs by enzymatically breaking the four membered ring. These drugs are effective against some gram negative cocci, but they are inactive against gram negative bacilli.

Group III includes ampicillin and amoxicillin; they are known as the "amino" penicillins because of the amino group on their side chains. This amino group makes them more hydrophilic, allowing them easier passage into gram-negative bacteria. They are effective against *Neisseria gonorrhoeae*, *Neisseria meningitidis*, *Haemophilus influenzae*, *E. coli*, *Listeria meningitis*, and *Proteus mirabilis*. Many bacteria are resistant to ampicillin and amoxicillin.

Amoxicillin is combined with clavulanic acid, (in tablet or suspension form) an inhibitor of beta-lactamases, to extend its spectrum of action. For hospitalized patients, ampicillin is commonly combined with sulbactam, another inhibitor of beta-lactamases; its spectrum of action is also extended with sulbactam. With clavulanic acid and sulbactam, both are more effective against bacteria producing beta-lactamases, including *S. aureus* and *Klebsiella*.

Group IV includes ticarcillin and piperacillin; they are broad spectrum antibiotics. Ticarcillin is commonly combined with clavulanic acid to increase its effectiveness and spectrum of action. Piperacillin is combined with tazobactam to extend its spectrum of action. They are effective against *Pseudomonas* and *Enterobacter*, both gram negative rods.

DRUG RESISTANCE

Bacteria develop resistance to antibiotics through a variety of mechanisms. Beta-lactamase, an enzyme that destroys beta-lactam drugs, confers resistance to bacteria producing it. A beta-lactam ring is essential for penicillins to work. Beta-lactamases break the bond between the carbonyl carbon and the nitrogen atom in the beta-lactam ring, rendering the drug useless. Gram positive and gram negative bacteria make

beta-lactamases.

Bacteria also resist beta-lactam drugs by changing the structure of transpeptidase and other PBPs, so drugs cannot inactivate transpeptidase or other PBPs.

SIDE-EFFECTS

Penicillins and cephalosporins are well tolerated. Most side-effects are limited to gastrointestinal problems such as diarrhea, nausea, and vomiting. Some people have hypersensitivity reactions to these drugs causing rashes, and, infrequently, anaphylactic reactions, which can be life-threatening. About, ten percent of patients develop hypersensitivity reactions. Penicillins can bind with human proteins, causing the immune system to consider the combined product to be an antigen.

Friendly gastrointestinal bacteria normally prevent harmful bacteria from growing. Antibiotics can substantially reduce friendly bacteria in the gastrointestinal tract, allowing harmful bacteria such as *clostridium difficile* to proliferate and harm the patient. *Clostridium difficile* is a serious infection, requiring treatment with other antibiotics.

DRUG INTERACTIONS

Some penicillins, amoxicillin, and ampicillin, etc., may increase methotrexate levels and warfarin levels. Increased methotrexate levels may be harmful to the patient; lowering methotrexate's dose may be necessary to avoid adverse effects. Increased warfarin levels may prolong bleeding. Deciding whether to lower a patient's warfarin dose should be made on a case by case basis.

CEPHALOSPORINS

Cephalosporins and penicillins are largely structurally quite similar, however, they differ in one important regard: the ring adjacent to the beta-lactam ring in penicillins has five members; the ring in cephalosporins has six members. This larger ring hinders beta-lactamase more than the five membered ring of penicillins. However, some bacteria have developed beta-lactamases that can break the beta lactam ring in cephalosporins.

Cephalosporins are classified according to generations. Presently, cephalosporins are divided into five generations. First generation cephalosporins are generally effective against gram positive bacteria such as *S. aureus*, *S. epidermidis*, *Streptococcus pyogenes* (group

A beta-hemolytic), *S. agalactiae*, and *S. pneumoniae* and some gram negative bacteria. Second generation cephalosporins are more effective against gram negative bacteria (*Haemophilus influenzae*) than the first generation cephalosporins. Third generation cephalosporins are considered to be broad spectrum, but they have broader coverage relative to gram negative than gram positive. The fourth generation cephalosporin cefepime has good coverage against *E. coli*, *Haemophilus influenzae*, and *Pseudomonas aeruginosa*. Ceftaroline, a fifth generation cephalosporin, is effective against methicillin-resistant *S. aureus* and vancomycin resistant *S. aureus*.

SIDE-EFFECTS

Most cephalosporins are well tolerated and only a small percentage of patients experience side-effects necessitating withdrawal. As with penicillins, patients can develop hypersensitivity reactions to cephalosporins. These reactions include anaphylaxis, bronchospasm, and urticaria. Cefotetan can cause bleeding, thrombocytopenia, and a prolonged PT. Consequently, monitor patients who are receiving anticoagulant medications. In addition, as with most antibiotics, diarrhea is a common side-effect. In rare instances, cephalosporins have caused fatal hemolysis. Some cases of nephrotoxicity have occurred.

INHIBITORS OF PROTEIN SYNTHESIS

Aminoglycosides, lincosamides, macrolides, tetracyclines, streptogramins, chloramphenicol, and oxazolidinone disrupt protein synthesis by inhibiting bacterial ribosomes. Ribosomes make proteins. Bacterial ribosomes have two main subunits, the "30S subunit" and the "50S subunit." The names 30S and 50S describe their molecular weight. These subunits are further divided into even smaller subunits. The 30S subunit and the 50S subunit together make up the ribosome. Any molecule disrupting either the 30s or 50S subunit or the interface between these units inhibits protein synthesis. Aminoglycosides, tetracycline, and tetracycline derivatives bind to the 30S ribosomal subunit and block protein synthesis. Chloramphenicol, macrolides, lincosamides, streptogramins, and oxazolidinone all block parts of the 50s subunit to block protein synthesis.

AMINOGLYCOSIDES

Aminoglycosides are principally used against aerobic gram negative bacteria. Common gram negative bacteria include *Escherichia coli*, *Klebsiella pneumoniae*, *Proteus mirabilis*, and *Pseudomonas aeruginosa*. Aminoglycosides are used with penicillins to treat bacterial endocarditis caused by gram positive bacteria. For patients with cystic fibrosis, tobramycin is used to treat lung infections caused by *Pseudomonas aeruginosa*. Aminoglycosides are generally ineffective against anaerobic bacteria because aminoglycosides depend on oxygen for entry into the bacteria.

Aminoglycosides bind with the 30S ribosomal subunit. They have three mechanisms of action: 1) disrupting the start of protein synthesis; 2) incorporating the wrong amino acid into a protein, thus making the protein useless; and 3) stopping protein synthesis before it normally would, thus creating an incomplete and useless protein.

Aminoglycosides are poorly absorbed from the GI tract; for systemic infections, aminoglycosides must be administered intramuscularly or intravenously. Renal impairment requires decreased doses. As creatine clearance decreases, the dose of the aminoglycoside must decrease as well to avoid toxicity.

Bacteria resist aminoglycosides through three main mechanisms: 1) altering the ribosome's structure so drugs cannot bind with it; 2) inactivating enzymes (similar to beta-lactamases); and 3) altering water-channels, preventing aminoglycosides from entering the bacteria.

SIDE-EFFECTS

Side-effects include ototoxicity and renal toxicity. Ototoxicity (hearing loss) is usually permanent. Patients should be warned to monitor for ringing in the ears, a signal of ensuing ear damage. Aminoglycosides also cause renal impairment, that if caught early, can be reversed. Serum concentrations of aminoglycosides must be checked to protect patients against adverse effects. If necessary, hemodialysis and peritoneal dialysis can remove aminoglycosides.

DRUG INTERACTIONS

Several drugs may aggravate renal toxicity. These drugs include amphotericin B, angiotensin converting enzyme inhibitors, cyclosporin, furosemide, thiazide diuretics, triamterene, NSAIDs, sulfonamides, and vancomycin. If possible, use another drug, if not, a dose reduction must be made to avoid nephrotoxicity.

Aminoglycosides are not susceptible to drug interactions involving the CYP system.

LINCOSAMIDES

Clindamycin (bacteriostatic) binds with the 50S subunit, preventing protein synthesis. Clindamycin is used for anaerobic bacteria, including *Bacteroides fragilis*. It is commonly used for dental infections, facial acne and bacterial vaginosis.

Clindamycin, by destroying friendly GI bacteria, allows *Clostridium difficile* to grow, causing pseudomembranous colitis. Clindamycin causes this problem more frequently than other antibiotics. Treat it with oral metronidazole or oral vancomycin. Consequently, use another effective antibiotic when available. Also, clindamycin has caused Stevens-Johnson Syndrome. Instruct patients to immediately stop the medication at the first sign of an allergic response.

Clindamycin and erythromycin prevent each other from fully working; they should not be used together.

MACROLIDES

The macrolides (bacteriostatic) include erythromycin, clarithromycin, and azithromycin. They bind with the 50S subunit, preventing newly formed proteins from leaving the ribosome. Erythromycin is effective against aerobic gram positive cocci including *streptococcus pyogenes* and penicillin-susceptible *streptococcus pneumoniae*. It is also effective against *H. influenzae* and *N. meningitidis*.

Telithromycin, a ketolide drug, is similar in structure to the macrolides. Telithromycin blocks the 50S ribosomal subunit, preventing protein synthesis. Bacteria are less resistant to telithromycin than erythromycin. It is effective against *Streptococcus pneumoniae*.

Erythromycin causes substantial gastrointestinal upset; this is the reason why it has so many different formulations. Erythromycin rarely causes substantial liver problems.

Erythromycin is a potent inhibitor of CYP 3A4. It inhibits the metabolism of carbamazepine, digoxin, theophylline, and warfarin.

TETRACYCLINES

The tetracycline class includes tetracycline itself, doxycycline, minocycline, and tigecycline. They inhibit protein synthesis by binding to the 30S ribosomal subunit. They are broad spectrum antibiotics effective against both gram positive and gram negative bacteria. Tigecycline treats complicated skin and skin structure infections (*Bacteroides fragilis*, *Streptococcus pyogenes*), complicated intra-abdominal infections (*E. coli*, *Klebsiella pneumoniae*), and community-acquired bacterial pneumonia (*Streptococcus pneumoniae*, *Haemophilus influenzae*, and *Legionella pneumophila*).

Bacteria resist tetracyclines by actively pumping tetracyclines out. They also produce enzymes that inactivate tetracyclines, same concept as beta-lactamases. Finally, bacteria alter the structure of the ribosome where tetracyclines bind to resist these drugs.

Tetracyclines adversely affect the kidneys. Kidney problems may necessitate switching to a different drug. Tetracyclines also cause gastrointestinal side-effects, similar to other antibiotics. Tetracyclines can discolor teeth.

Tetracyclines bind with calcium ions in the gastrointestinal tract, limiting their absorption; space them by at least two hours.

CHLORAMPHENICOL

Chloramphenicol (broad spectrum, bacteriostatic) binds with the 50S subunit, blocking protein synthesis. It works against both gram positive and gram negative bacteria (aerobic and anaerobic). Although it is broad spectrum, it is a last choice for many infections such as typhoid fever because of severe adverse effects resulting from inhibiting human protein synthesis.

STREPTOGRAMINS

Dalfopristin, a group A streptogramin, and, quinupristin, a group B streptogramin, are combined in one dosage form. Dalfopristin/quinupristin was specially FDA approved to treat life-threatening infections caused by *Enterococcus faecium*; it also treats *Staphylococcus aureus*, and *Streptcoccus pyogenes*. Dalfopristin inhibits the early phase of protein synthesis. Quinupristin inhibits the late phase of protein synthesis. Both bind with the 23S rRNA of the 50S ribosomal subunit.

It significantly inhibits CYP450 3A4, increasing levels of cyclosporin A, midazolam, and nifedipine. It can inhibit the metabolism of drugs that cause QT prolongation. It has not been shown to interfere with the functioning of other antibiotics.

Dalfopristin/quinupristin has caused *Clostridi-*

um difficile associated diarrhea.

After administering dalfopristin/quinupristin, flush the vein with 5% Dextrose in Water; do not flush with saline or heparin because of incompatibility.

OXAZOLIDINONE

Linezolid binds to the 23S ribosomal RNA of the 50S subunit, preventing protein synthesis. It is effective against a wide-range of gram positive bacteria including vancomycin resistant *Enterococcus faecium*, *Staphylococcus aureus* (including methicillin resistant strains), *Streptococcus pneumoniae*, *Streptcoccus pyogenes*, and *Streptococcus agalactiae*.

Monitor complete blood counts weekly. Linezolid has caused myelosuppression (anemia, leukopenia, pancytopenia, and thrombocytopenia). Consider discontinuing linezolid in patients who develop these conditions or a pre-existing condition worsens.

Linezolid can cause hypoglycemia in patients receiving insulin or oral hypoglycemic drugs.

TOPOISOMERASE INHIBITORS

Quinolone antibiotics prevent the enzyme "type II topoisomerase" from assisting with DNA replication. During DNA replication, type II topoisomerases perform two main functions. First, they uncoil DNA supercoils- DNA naturally exists in a supercoil shape that must be relaxed so the necessary enzymes can replicate it. Second, after replication, the two DNA copies (each copy has two strands, four strands total) must be separated from each other, so one copy can go to one daughter cell and the other copy can go to the other daughter cell- type II topoisomerase does this.

The newer fluoroquinolones (a subset of the quinolones) are more commonly used; they have a fluorine atom which enhances their antibacterial activity. The fluoroquinolones include norfloxacin, ciprofloxacin, ofloxacin, gemifloxacin, levofloxacin, and moxifloxacin. They are effective against respiratory tract infections, acute sinusitis, urinary tract infections, opthalmic infection, and ear infections. They are effective against gram-negative bacteria such as *Klebsiella pneumoniae*, *Escherichia coli*, *Proteus mirabilis*, and *Haemophilus influenzae*. The older quinolones are rarely used today.

Few patients experience nausea, vomiting, and diarrhea. Fluoroquinolones can cause tendinopathy and tendon rupture. The Achilles tendon is most frequently affected, but tendons in the thumb, hand, biceps, and rotator cuff have also been affected. Fluo-

roquinolones can prolong the QT interval; avoid using them in patients with known prolongation of the QT interval.

Ciprofloxacin inhibits CYP1A2. The co-administration of ciprofloxacin and theophylline has been fatal; avoid using them together.

Antacids, particularly calcium, prevent the absorption of quinolones.

INHIBITORS OF RNA SYNTHESIS

Rifabutin and rifampin prevent the transcription of DNA to RNA by inhibiting the enzyme RNA Polymerase. This prevents functional RNA from reaching the ribosomes. Ribosomes use RNA as a blueprint for protein production.

Rifabutin inhibits RNA Polymerase in *Escherichia coli* and *Bacillus subtilis*. Rifampin inhibits RNA Polymerase in susceptible strains of *Mycobacterium tuberculosis* and *Neisseria meningitidis*. Rifampin also has *in vitro* activity against *Staphylococcus aureus* and *Staphylococcus epidermidis*.

Rifampin is mainly used for tuberculosis; it must be used with other antibiotics to limit resistance development. Rifampin, isoniazid, and pyrazinamide are used together for two months as initial therapy to treat tuberculosis.

Rifabutin induces CYP3A4 isoenzymes. It lowers blood levels of itraconazole, dapsone, sulfamethoxazole-trimethoprim, delavirdine, nelfinavir, and clarithromycin.

Rifampin is contraindicated in patients being treated with ritonavir-boosted saquinavir because the risk of severe hepatocellular toxicity increases. Rifampin reduces blood levels of most HIV antiviral drugs.

Bacteria develop resistance by changing the structure of RNA Polymerase so these drugs cannot bind to it.

ANTIMETABOLITES

Bacteria need folic acid to produce DNA. Bacteria must manufacture folic acid; they cannot absorb it from the environment. Folic acid is used to build purines and pyrimidines- the building blocks of DNA. Bacteria depend on the enzymes dihydropteroate synthase and dihydrofolate reductase to produce folic acid. If dihydropteroate synthase and/or dihydrofolate reductase are inhibited, then bacteria cannot produce the building blocks of DNA.

Sulfamethoxazole and sulfadiazine (sulfon-

amides) inhibit dihydropteroate synthase. Trimethoprim inhibits dihydrofolate reductase. Sulfonamides
and trimethoprim are bacteriostatic.

Sulfamethoxazole and trimethoprim are combined into one tablet (Bactrim™, or Septra®) to syner-
gistically treat infections. Besides treating uncompli-
cated urinary tract infections, salmonella, and typhoid
fever, it also treats pneumocystis jiroveci pneumonia,
a common infection in immunocompromised patients.

Sulfamethoxazole and/or sulfadiazine can cause
Stevens-Johnson Syndrome, toxic epidermal necrolysis,
fulminant hepatic necrosis, agranulocytosis, aplastic
anemia, and other blood dyscrasias.

Sulfamethoxazole and trimethoprim can cause
Clostridium difficile associated diarrhea. Further, sulfamethoxazole and trimethoprim can increase warfarin's
anticoagulant action.

Antibiotics that Lyse Bacteria by Disrupting the Cell Wall				
Generic Name/ Brand Name	Clinical Use	Dose	Mechanism of Action	Dosage Form
Natural Penicillins				
Penicillin VK	Penicillin sensitive *S. Aureus*	500 mg three times daily	Inhibits peptide cross-linking preventing cell wall synthesis	Tablets 250 mg, 500 mg, Suspension
Penicillin G Benza-thine Bicillin® L-A	Syphilis, yaws, Group A Streptococcal, prophylaxis for rheu-matic fever	1.2 Million Units as a single dose	Same as above	IM, Do NOT administer IV
Penicillin G Benza-thine and Penicillin G Procaine/ Bicillin® C-R, Bicil-lin® C-R 900/300	Group A Streptococ-cal, Pneumococcal infections,	2.4 Million Units in a single dose	Same as above	IM, Do NOT administer IV
Penicillinase-Resistant Penicillins: *Staphylococcus aureus* and *Staphylococcus epidermidis*				
Dicloxacillin Dycill	Methicillin sensitive *S. Aureus* and *S. epidermidis*	Adults 250-1000 mg every 6 hours	Altered chemical structure reduces susceptibility to beta-lactamase	Capsules 250 mg and 500 mg
Nafcillin	Same as above	IM 500 mg every 4 to 6 hours, IV 500-2000 mg ev-ery 4 to 6 hours	Same as above	IM, IV
Oxacillin	Same as above	Adults IM 250-2000 mg every 4 to 6 hours	Same as above	IM, IV

Antibiotics that Lyse Bacteria by Disrupting the Cell Wall				
Generic Name/ Brand Name	Clinical Use	Dose	Mechanism of Action	Dosage Form
Aminopenicillins: Mainly used against susceptible gram negative bacteria *H. influenzae, E.coli, Proteus Mirabilis*; Gram positive *Staphylococcus aureus, Streptococcus pneumoniae*				
Amoxicillin Amoxil®	Otitis media due to *S. aureus*, and *S. pneumoniae*	500 mg three times daily	Same as above	Tablets 875 mg, Capsules 250 mg, 500 mg, IV
Amoxicillin/Clavulanate Potassium Augmentin®	Same as above	500 mg three times daily	Same as above	Tablets 500 mg, 875 mg, 1000 mg
Ampicillin Principen®	Same as above	Oral, IM, or IV 250-500 every 6 hours	Same as above. This subclass of drugs has an "amino" group, making them water soluble enough to pass through the porins in gram negative bacteria.	Capsules 250 mg and 500 mg; IM, IV

Antibiotics that Lyse Bacteria by Disrupting the Cell Wall				
Extended Spectrum Penicillins Anti-Pseudomonas				
Generic Name/ Brand Name	Clinical Use	Dose	Mechanism of Action	Dosage Form
Piperacillin and Tazobactam Zosyn®	Respiratory infections and urinary tract infections due to susceptible strains of *Pseudomonas, Proteus, E. Coil,*	Adults IV 3.375 gms every 6 hours. For nosocomial pneumonia start at 4.5 grams every 6 hours	Inhibits peptide cross-linking preventing cell wall synthesis	IV
Ticarcillin Clavulanate Timentin®	*Enterobacter* infections; Lower respiratory tract infections: caused by susceptible strains of *Pseudomonas, H. influenzae, Klebsiella, Staphylococcus,* and *Serratia*	Septicemia and UTI: 3.1 grams every 4 to 6 hours	Same as above	IV

First Generation Cephalosporins: gram positive cocci *S. aureus, S. epidermidis, Streptococcus pyogenes* (group A beta-hemolytic), *S. agalactiae, S. pneumoniae*				
Generic Name/ Brand Name	Clinical Use	Usual Dose	Pharmacokinetics	Dosage Form
Cefadroxil Duricef®	Active against gram positive cocci; limited against gram negative bacteria. Infections due to *Streptococcus pyogenes, S. pneumoniae*	Uncomplicated UTI: 1 gram to 2 grams in one to two divided doses. Other UTI: 1 gram twice daily	Near complete oral absorption	Capsules 500mg, tablets 1 gram, suspension 250 mg/5ml and 500 mg/5ml

Cefazolin Ancef®	Staphylococcal endocarditis caused by methicillin susceptible strains. Bone and joint infections caused by *Staphylococcus aureus*. Respiratory tract infections from susceptible strains of *S. pneumoniae, S. pyogenes, S. aureus, Klebsiella,* or *H. influenzae*	Mild infections: 250 mg to 500 mg every 8 hours. Moderate: 500 mg to 1000 mg every 6 to 8 hours. Severe: 1 gram to 1.5 grams every 6 hours	Poor oral absorption. Administered IV or IM	Solution
Cephalexin Keflex®	Respiratory tract infections due to *S. pneumoniae*, otitis media, skin and skin structure infections, urinary tract infections	250 mg to 1000 mg four times daily for most infections.	Good oral absorption	Capsules 250 mg and 500 mg

Second Generation Cephalosporins: Haemophilus influenzae and generally same coverage as first generation				
Generic Name/ Brand Name	Clinical Use	Dose	Mechanism of Action	Dosage Form
Cefaclor/ Ceclor	Acute otitis media from *Streptococcus pneumoniae, H. influenzae, S. pyogenes*. Respiratory tract infections from susceptible *S. pneumoniae,* or *H. infleunzae,*	250 mg orally every 8 hours	Inhibits peptide cross-linking preventing cell wall synthesis	Capsules 250 mg and 500 mg; Suspension
Cefotetan/ Cefotan	Urinary tract infection from *E. coli*	1 gm - 2 gm once daily; doses vary depending on infection	Same as above	Injection (powder for reconstitution) 1 gm, 2 gm, 10 gm
Cefoxitin/ Mefoxin®	Lower respiratory tract infections from *S. pneumoniae*	1 gm every 6 to 8 hours, doses vary depending on infection	Same as above	Injection vials (powder for reconstitution) 1 gm, 2 gm, 10 gm

Second Generation Cephalosporins: Haemophilus influenzae and generally same coverage as first generation				
Cefuroxime/ Ceftin®	Otitis media *S. from pyogenes, S. pneumoniae, or H. influenzae.* Ear, nose, throat infections *H. influenzae,*	250 mg - 500 mg twice daily	Same as above	Tablet 250 mg and 500 mg; Suspension 125 mg/5ml; 250 mg/5ml

Third Generation Cephalosporins Broad Spectrum: Mostly gram negative but some gram positive				
Generic Name/ Brand Name	Clinical Use	Dose	Mechanism of Action	Dosage Form
Cefotaxime Claforan®	Lower respiratory tract infections, urinary tract infections, gynecologic infections. Gonorrhea.	600 mg -1000 mg every 8 to 12 Hours IV	Inhibits peptide cross-linking preventing cell wall synthesis	Injection (powder for reconstitution) 500 mg, 1 gm, 2 gm, 10 gm
Ceftazidime Fortaz®	Lower respiratory tract infections, skin and skin structure infections, urinary tract infections, bacterial septicemia, bone and joint infections.	1 gm every 8 to 12 hours	Same as above	Injection (powder for reconstitution) 1 gm, 2 gm, 6 gm vials
Ceftriaxone Rocephin®	Lower respiratory tract infections from *S. pneumoniae, S. aureus, H. influenzae.* Gonorrhea.	50 mg-300 mg three times daily	Same as above	Injection (powder for reconstitution) 250 mg, 500 mg, 1 gm, 2 gm, 10 gm vials
Fourth Generation Cephalosporin				
Cefepime Maxipime™	Infections caused by *E. coli, Haemophilus influenzae,* and *Pseudomonas aeruginosa*	1 gm - 2 gm every 12 hours	Same as above	Injection (powder for reconstitution) 500 mg, 1 gm, 2 gm

Tetracycline Derivatives: Inhibiting the 30S Ribosomal Subunit, Inhibiting Protein Synthesis				
Generic Name/ Brand Name	Clinical Use	Dose	Mechanism of Action	Dosage Form
Doxycycline Hyclate/ Vibramycin®, Monodox®	Respiratory tract infections from *Mycoplasma pneumoniae,* Chlamydia, Rickettsiae	100 mg Bid to Tid	Binds to the 30s subunit blocking tRNA from transferring bacterial amino-acids.	Tablets, Capsules 50 mg and 100 mg (many others)
Minocycline/ Minocin®	Same as above, also used for acne	50-100 mg QD to BID	Same as above.	Tablets and Capsules 50 mg, 75 mg, 100 mg; Injection (powder for reconstitution) 100 mg vial
Tetracycline/	Same as above, also used for acne	250-500 mg Bid	Same as above.	Capsules 250 mg and 500 mg; Suspension

Macrolides: Inhibiting the 50S Ribosomal Subunit				
Generic Name/ Brand Name	Clinical Use	Dose	Mechanism of Action	Dosage Form
Azithromycin/ Zithromax®	Community acquired pneumonia caused by *Chlamydia pneumoniae*, *H. influenzae*, *Moraxella catarrhalis*, Pelvic inflammatory disease caused by *Chlamydia trachomatis*	500 mg on day 1, 250 mg on days 2 to 4	Binds with 50S subunit preventing protein synthesis.	Azithromycin 250 mg tablets (pack of 6). Suspension 100 mg/5ml , 200 mg/5ml
Clarithromycin/ Biaxin®	Used in combination with lansoprazole and amoxicillin for *H. pylori*, acute otitis media caused by *H. influenzae*, *Moraxella catarrhalis*, or *Streptococcus pneumoniae*	250-500 mg BID	Same as above.	Tablets 250 mg and 500 mg; Suspension 125 mg/5ml, 250 mg /5ml both in 50 ml and 100 ml bottles
Erythromycin Ethylsuccinate/ E.E.S.®	Upper and lower respiratory tract infections caused by *S. pyogenes* and *S. pneumoniae*	400 mg Tid	Same as above.	E.E.S. 400 mg tablet
Chloramphenicol	Typhoid fever	50-100 mg/kg/ day in divided doses Q6H	Same as above.	IV

Lincosamides: Inhibiting the 50S Ribosomal Subunit				
Generic Name/ Brand Name	Clinical Use	Dose	Mechanism of Action	Dosage Form
Clindamycin/ Cleocin®	Bacterial vaginosis (*Haemophilus* vaginitis, *Gardnerella* vaginitis, *Corynebacterium* vaginitis); *Bacteroides fragilis*; acne	150-300 mg TID	Prevents protein synthesis by binding with 50S ribosomal subunit	Capsules 150 mg and 300; Gel, Suspension, Vaginal Ovules, IV
Oxazolidiones: Inhibiting the 50S Ribosomal Subunit				
Linezolid/ Zyvox®	Vancomycin resistant *Enterococcus faecium*	600 mg Q12H for 10-14 days	Binds to the 23S ribosomal RNA of the 50s Subunit preventing protein synthesis	Tablets 600 mg; IV, infusion bag 200 mg /100 ml; Suspension 100 mg/5ml 150 ml bottle

Fluoroquinolones: Topoisomerase Inhibitors

Generic Name/ Brand Name	Clinical Use	Dose	Dosage Form
Ciprofloxacin/ Cipro ®XR	Uncomplicated urinary tract infections caused by E. coli, Proteus mirabilis, vancomycin-susceptible Enterococcus faecalis, or Staphylococcus saprophyticus; Complicated urinary tract infections caused by E. coli, K. pneumoniae, vancomycin-susceptible Enterococcus faecalis, P. mirabilis, or Pseudomonas aeruginosa	500 mg BID	Cipro ®XR just in tablets. Other formulations include oral suspension, opthalmic drops, ophthalmic ointment
Gatifloxacin / Zymar®	Bacterial conjunctivitis from susceptible strains of Staphylococcus aureus, Staphylococcus epidermidis, Streptococcus pneumoniae, Haemophilus influenzae	Days 1-2 1gtt AE Q2H while awake, Days 3-7 1gtt in AE QID	Opthalmic solution
Gemifloxacin/ Factive®	Acute bacterial exacerbation of chronic bronchitis due to Streptococcus pneumoniae, H. influenzae, H. parainfluenzae, or Moraxella catarrhalis; Community-acquired pneumonia due to S. pneumoniae (including multi-drug resistant strains), H. influenzae, M. catarrhalis, Mycoplasma pneumoniae, Chlamydia pneumoniae, Klebsiella pneumoniae.	320 mg QD	Tablet
Levofloxacin/ Levaquin®	Nosocomial and community acquired pneumonia, acute bacterial sinusitis, acute bacterial exacerbation of chronic bronchitis, skin and skin structure infections, chronic bacterial prostatitis, complicated and uncomplicated urinary tract infections, due to susceptible bacteria. Susceptible bacteria include Pseudomonas aeruginosa, E. coli, Klebsiella pneumoniae, H. influenzae, S. pneumoniae, Moraxella catarrhalis, and S. aureus.	Doses vary based on infection. 500 mg to 750 mg daily for 7 to 14 days.	Tablets, IV
Moxifloxacin/ Avelox®, Vigamox®	Avelox® is approved for acute bacterial sinusitis, acute bacterial exacerbation of chronic bronchitis, community acquired pneumonia, complicated and uncomplicated skin and skin structure infections, complicated intrabdominal infections. Susceptible bacteria include Streptococcus pneumoniae, H. influenzae, Moraxella catarrhalis, S. aureus, and E. coli.	400 mg QD for 5 to 14 days depending on infection.	Avelox® tablets Vigamox® Opthalmic drops

Anti-Metabolites				
Generic Name/ Brand Name	Clinical Use	Dose	Mechanism of Action	Dosage Form
Sulfadiazine	Toxoplasmosis	Toxoplasmosis patients <60 kg 1000 mg q6h for a minimum of 6 weeks. Patients >60 kg 1500 mg q6h for a minimum of 6 weeks	Inhibits dihydropteroate synthase	500 mg tablet
Trimethoprim/Sulfamethoxazole / Bactrim™, Bactrim™ DS, Septra®, Septra® DS	Uncomplicated urinary tract infections, salmonella, typhoid fever, and pneumocystis jiroveci pneumonia	Most infections, one double strength tablet twice daily. No alcohol.	Trimethoprim inhibits dihydrofolate reductase. Sulfamethoxazole inhibits dihydropteroate synthase.	Tablets: trimethoprim 80 mg and sulfa. 400 mg; and double strength trimethoprim 160 mg and sulfa. 800 mg

CHAPTER 23

ANTIVIRAL MEDICATIONS

Viruses have multiple steps in their life cycle. Antiviral medications prevent these steps from occurring; thus preventing viruses from growing. Viral replication, in general, includes the following steps: attaching to the cell, entering the cell, removing the coating over its DNA or RNA (viruses have either DNA or RNA), replicating its DNA or RNA, producing the proteins it needs, assembling new viruses, and then exiting the cell. Antiviral medications exist that prevent each of these steps. HIV viruses must change their RNA into DNA with reverse transcription enzymes so the newly formed viral DNA can enter the cell's nucleus where it is incorporated into human DNA and then undergoes transcription back into RNA.

HERPES MEDICATIONS

The principal drugs in this section are acyclovir, valacyclovir, penciclovir, and famciclovir. Acyclovir is representative of this group. Acyclovir treats both herpes simplex virus-1 and herpes simplex virus-2. Acyclovir treats various manifestations of herpes including herpes encephalitis, genital herpes, eye infections caused by herpes, and neonatal herpes simplex infections, which is a serious infection in newborns. Acyclovir is used to treat varicella-zoster infections in immunocompetent patients who may be at risk of moderate to severe varicella and for immunocompromised patients. Further, acyclovir substantially decreases the severity of herpes zoster infections in immunocompetent adults; it is also used for herpes zoster in immuno-compromised patients.

Acyclovir is generally well tolerated in most patients. However, it can cause injection site reactions including inflammation or phlebitis. It can cause anemia and thrombocytopenia. It may cause renal dysfunction, especially in patients who are dehydrated. It can be administered without regard for food.

These drugs prevent the herpes virus from replicating its DNA. Acyclovir, famciclovir, and penciclovir are three nucleoside analog anti-herpes drugs (famciclovir is metabolized to penciclovir; valacyclovir is a prodrug for acyclovir). Nucleosides have two main mechanisms of action. First, they inhibit DNA Polymerases by competing with normal nucleotide bases

(deoxyguanosine triphosphate) for incorporation into a growing strand of DNA. Second, nucleoside analogs, after incorrect incorporation into a growing strand of DNA, prevent DNA Polymerases from adding the next DNA base pair, thus stopping growth of the DNA strand. These drugs are shaped in such a way that the next DNA base pair cannot be physically attached to the drug, hence the DNA strand stops growing. This same principle is used in HIV antiviral medications. These drugs, after being incorporated into a growing DNA strand, may prevent the release of DNA polymerase. These drugs have to be metabolized inside infected cells to their respective triphosphate forms. Viral cells use the enzyme thymidine kinase to convert acyclovir to acyclovir monophosphate. Other enzymes then convert it to the diphosphate and triphosphate forms. DNA base pairs are all triphosphates. Non-infected cells do not convert acyclovir to its triphosphate form, and, hence, it does not harm non-infected cells.

COMMON COLD MEDICATIONS

Amantadine and rimantidine treat influenza A infections. Amantadine and rimantadine prevent viral RNA from being uncoated, which necessarily prevents its reproduction. Amantadine and rimantadine block ion channels (M2 matrix protein), preventing acid from dissolving the final coating protecting viral RNA. They decrease the symptoms one experiences while suffering from the common cold. They are less expensive than oseltamivir and zanamivir. Amantadine and rimantadine are chemically classified as adamantanes. Some strains of influenza A are resistant to amantadine and rimantadine (H3N2, H1N1).

Amantadine causes anticholinergic side-effects that are dose-dependent, as the dose increases, the severity of side-effects increase. Amantadine has caused death at as little as 1 gram, which is just ten of the standard strength capsules or tablets. Amantadine overdoses affect the heart, respiratory systems, kidneys, and CNS. Suicide attempts have happened in patients taking amantadine.

Oseltamivir and zanamivir are effective against both influenza A and influenza B viruses. They inhibit the release of newly formed viruses from human cells. They competitively and reversibly block the enzyme neuraminidase from cutting the newly formed viruses free from their host cell. Because they are specific to viral enzymes, they cause little harm to human cells.

Oseltamivir is administered orally at 75 mg twice daily for 5 days for adult doses to treat infections. For prophylaxis it is dosed at 75 mg once daily for 10 days when others in the home have influenza. For effectiveness, these medications must be started within two days of developing symptoms of the common cold. They reduce infection by 1 to 1.5 days.

Oseltamivir has caused Stevens-Johnson Syndrome; caution patients to discontinue use if an allergic like reaction occurs. The medical provider should counsel patients to watch for signs of an allergic reaction. Oseltamivir can cause patients to experience abnormal behavior. The most common adverse reactions are nausea and vomiting.

Zanamivir is administered by inhalation only. It is dosed at 10 mg twice daily for 5 days in adults and children older than 7. It can worsen asthma; otherwise, it is well tolerated.

Just as bacteria develop resistance to antibiotics, viruses develop resistance to antiviral medications. Influenza can develop resistance by physically changing the enzyme neuraminidase so these drugs do not inhibit it.

HIV MEDICATIONS

FUSION PROTEIN INHIBITORS

Maraviroc and enfuvirtide prevent the HIV-1 virus from attaching to and entering human cells. Certain molecules on HIV-1's outer coating must bind with certain receptors on human cells before HIV-1 can enter human cells. Gp120 is the molecule on HIV-1's surface that must bind with the human cell receptor called "CCR5" before HIV-1 can enter human cells. Maraviroc is a CCR5 co-receptor antagonist. It binds with the CCR5 receptor, preventing the binding of HIV-1 gp120 to CCR5, thus preventing the entry of "CCR5-tropic HIV-1" into human cells. HIV has several different forms; maraviroc does not work against "CXCR-tropic HIV-1" and "dual-tropic HIV-1."

Enfuvirtide is an HIV-1 fusion inhibitor; it inhibits the fusion of human cell membranes with HIV-1 membranes (the outer envelope), thus prevent-ing HIV-1 from attaching to and entering human cells. HIV-1 membranes are in part made of glycoprotein. Glycoprotein 41 (gp-41) is an integral part of HIV-1 membranes. Two critical pieces of gp-41 are heptad-repeat-1 (HR-1) and heptad-repeat-2 (HR-2). HR-1 and HR-2 must bind with each other before HIV-1 can enter human cells. Enfuvirtide binds with HR-1 preventing HR1- from binding with HR-2; thus preventing HIV-1 from entering human cells. Resistance to enfuvirtide occurs by alteration of the enfuvirtide's binding site. Enfuvirtide must be used in combination with other drugs to decrease the development of resistance.

Patients using enfuvirtide are more likely to develop bacterial pneumonia than they would otherwise. Injection site reactions, diarrhea, and nausea are common adverse reactions.

Dosage adjustment is not necessary in patients with impaired renal function. Enfuvirtide does not cause any known interaction with the CYP450 system.

NUCLEOSIDE ANALOG REVERSE TRANSCRIPTASE INHIBITORS

Zidovudine, lamivudine, stavudine, zalcitabine, emtricitabine, didanosine, and abacavir are nucleoside analog reverse transcriptase inhibitors. Their physical structure allows them to be incorporated into a growing DNA strand. They inhibit the enzyme reverse transcriptase by ending DNA chain growth after being incorrectly added by reverse transcriptase into a DNA chain. After being incorrectly added to a growing DNA chain, their physical structure prevents reverse transcriptase from adding the next nucleotide; hence reverse transcriptase is inhibited. All of these drugs have to be phosphorylated before they can be incorporated into DNA (the phosphate bonds of DNA are integral to its structure). Tenofovir is a nucleotide analogue reverse transcriptase inhibitor of reverse transcriptase. It already has the necessary phosphate group needed for incorporation into a new strand of DNA. It also ends DNA chain growth.

NON-NUCLEOSIDE REVERSE TRANSCRIPTASE INHIBITORS

Non-nucleoside reverse transcriptase inhibitors directly inhibit reverse transcriptase without having to be incorporated into a growing DNA chain. They bind directly with reverse transcriptase near the site where a nucleotide base pair would bind. They physically prevent the transfer of the nucleotide base pair to the growing DNA chain, thus ending growth of that chain. These drugs include delavirdine, efavirenz, etravirine, and nevirapine.

Delavirdine is contraindicated with alprazolam, midazolam, and triazolam because it substantially increases their blood levels by decreasing their metabolism through CYP3A enzymes. It is also contraindicated with ergot derivatives and pimozide.

Efavirenz can cause severe depression and/or suicidal ideation. Liver function tests need to be monitored before and during treatment in patients with hepatic diseases, including hepatitis B or C, marked transaminase elevations, and patients who are taking drugs that may cause liver toxicity. Efavirenz should not be used as a single agent or added as a single agent to a failing regimen.

PROTEASE INHIBITORS

Multiple HIV-1 protease inhibitors have been developed; they include amprenavir, atazanavir, darunavir, fosamprenavir, indinavir, lopinavir, nelfinavir, ritonavir, saquinavir, and tipranavir. All inhibit the enzyme HIV protease from cleaving proteins to their final and functional sizes; that is HIV proteins remain in non-functional states. HIV protease cleaves proteins to their final length, including reverse transcriptase (without HIV protease, HIV cannot produce reverse transcriptase).

Ritonavir is a potent inhibitor of CYP450 3A most of the time (unusually, ritonavir sometimes induces CYP450 3A). Ritonavir increases trazodone levels several fold. Ritonavir substantially increases blood levels of colchicine; patients with renal or hepatic impairment should not receive colchicine with ritonavir. Ritonavir substantially decreases theophylline levels.

INTEGRASE INHIBITOR

Raltegravir prevents the incorporation of HIV viral DNA into human DNA, which is a necessary step for HIV viral DNA reproduction. Specifically, it inhibits the enzyme HIV integrase. It is approved for use in combination with other HIV antiretroviral drugs. The adult dose is 400 mg twice daily, with or without food. It has been associated with myopathy and rhabdomyolysis; use caution in patients at risk of myopathy or rhabdomyolysis. Rifampin may decrease its plasma levels.

Antiviral Drugs for Herpes

Generic Name	Brand Name	Dose	Mechanism of Action	Dosage Form
Acyclovir	Zovirax®	Mucocutaneous 400 mg every 4 hours while awake, 5 times daily for 7 to 14 days.	Inhibits DNA Polymerase	Tablets, Suspension, Cream, Ointment, IV
Valacyclovir	Valtrex®	Genital HSV-2 1000 mg twice daily for 7 to 10 days for initial infection. For recurrent infections 500 mg twice daily for 3 days.	Inhibits DNA Polymerase	Tablets
Famciclovir	Famvir®	Genital herpes initial episode 250 mg 3 times daily for 7 days. Recurrent episodes 1 gram twice daily for 1 day or 125 mg twice daily for 5 days depending on patient	Inhibits viral DNA replication	Tablets
Penciclovir	Denavir®	Cold sores apply every 2 hours while awake for 4 hours	Inhibits DNA replication	Cream 1%

Fusion Protein Inhibitors Against HIV

Generic Name	Brand Name	Dose	Mechanism of Action	Dosage Form
Enfuvirtide	Fuzeon®	16 years and older 90 mg twice daily subcutaneously	Fusion Protein Inhibitor	Injection
Maraviroc	Selzentry®	150 mg to 600 mg twice daily depending on other drugs patient is on	Same as above	Tablets 150 mg and 300 mg

Antivirals for the Common Cold

Generic Name	Brand Name	Dose	Mechanism of Action	Dosage Form
Amantadine	Symmetrel®	Adult daily dose: 100 mg once to twice daily for 5 to 7 days. Children 1 to 9 years, 5 mg /kg daily for 5 to 7 days (max of 150 mg daily)	Prevents uncoating of Influenza A virus	Capsule 100 mg, Tablet 100 mg, Syrup 50 mg/5ml
Rimantidine	Flumadine®	People over 10 years: 100 mg twice daily for 5 to 7 days for adults	Inhibits the uncoating of Influenza A,	Tablet 100 mg, Syrup 50 mg/5ml

Antivirals for the Common Cold				
Generic Name	Brand Name	Dose	Mechanism of Action	Dosage Form
Ribavirin	Virazole®	6 grams reconstituted with 300 ml of sterile water and administered by aerosol for 12-18 hours for 3 to 7 days.	Active against respiratory syncytial virus (RSV), nucleoside analogue that inhibits synthesis of DNA and RNA nucleotides	Lyophilized powder
Zanamivir	Relenza®	2 inhalations (10 mg) once daily for 28 days, start within 5 days of symptoms	Inhibits influenza neuraminidase enzymes, inhibiting release of viral particles.	Powder inside of an inhaler
Oseltamivir	Tamiflu®	People 13 or older 75 mg twice daily for 10 days for treatment. For prophylaxis, 75 mg once daily for 10 days when others in home have influenza (adult doses). Children 1 to 12, 30 mg to 75 mg twice daily for treatment	Inhibits viral neuraminidase preventing viral release of new viruses	Capsule, Powder for oral suspension

Chronic Hepatitis B				
Generic Name	Brand Name	Dose	Mechanism of Action	Dosage Form
Adefovir	Hepsera®	10 mg once daily orally	Inhibits viral RNA-dependent DNA Polymerase thus preventing replication	Tablets 10 mg

Antivirals for Retroviruses				
HIV-1 Reverse Transcriptase Inhibitors				
Generic Name	Brand Name	Dose	Mechanism of Action	Dosage Form
Abacavir	Ziagen®	Adults 300 mg twice daily or 600 mg once daily	Nucleoside reverse transcriptase inhibitor	Ziagen Tablets 300 mg, Solution 20 mg/ml
Didanosine	Videx® EC	Adults Less than 60 kg = 125 mg twice daily; 60 kg or greater 200 mg twice daily	Inhibits HIV reverse transcriptase, thus blocking viral DNA synthesis	Capsule Delayed release 200 mg 250 mg, 400 mg, Powder for solution 2 gm, and 4 gm
Emtricitabine	Emtriva®	200 mg once daily of capsule, 240 mg of solution once daily	Interferes with HIV viral RNA-dependent DNA polymerase, inhibiting replication	Capsules 200 mg, Solution 10 mg/ml

Antivirals for Retroviruses				
HIV-1 Reverse Transcriptase Inhibitors				
Generic Name	Brand Name	Dose	Mechanism of Action	Dosage Form
Lamivudine	Epivir® (for HIV), Epivir-HBV® (for hepatitis B)	For HIV 150 mg twice daily or 300 mg once daily, use with at least 2 other drugs	Inhibits HIV reverse transcriptase	Epivir tablets 150 mg, 300 mg; Epivir-HBV 100 mg QD; Solution 10mg/ml
Stavudine	Zerit®	Adults less than 60 kg 30 mg every 12 hours; Adults 60 kg or greater 40 mg every 12 hours	Nucleoside reverse transcriptase inhibitor; also interferes with DNA Polymerase	Adults less than 60 kg 30 mg Q12H; Adults 60 kg or greater 40 mg Q12H
Tenofovir	Viread®	300 mg once daily	Nucleotide reverse transcriptase inhibitor	Tablet 300 mg
Zidovudine	Retrovir®	300mg twice daily	Interferes with HIV viral RNA-dependent DNA polymerase, inhibiting replication	Tablet 300mg, Capsule 100mg, Injection 10mg/ml, Syrup 50mg/5ml

Antivirals Non-Nucleoside Inhibitors of HIV Reverse Transcriptase (NNRTIs)				
Generic Name	Brand Name	Dose	Mechanism of Action	Dosage Form
Delavirdine	Rescriptor®	400 mg three times daily	Non-nucleoside reverse transcriptase inhibitor	Tablet 100 mg, 200 mg
Efavirenz	Sustiva®	Adult 600 mg once daily	Same as above	Tablet 600 mg, Capsule 50 mg, 100 mg
Etravirine	Intelence®	200 mg twice daily after meals. For patients who are resistant to delavirdine, efavirenz, or nevirapine	Same as above	
Nevirapine	Viramune®	Initial dose 200 mg once daily for 14 days then 200 mg twice daily; must use in combination	Same as above	Tablet 200 mg, Suspension 50 mg/5ml

Antivirals Protease Inhibitors Against HIV				
Generic Name	Brand Name	Dose	Mechanism of Action	Dosage Form
Amprenavir	Agenerase	Adults 1200 mg twice daily	Inhibits HIV Protease preventing infectious viral particles from forming	Capsule 50 mg

Antivirals Protease Inhibitors Against HIV				
Generic Name	Brand Name	Dose	Mechanism of Action	Dosage Form
Atanzanavir	Reyataz®	400 mg once daily	Same as above	Capsule 100 mg, 150 mg, 200 mg, 300 mg
Fosamprenavir	Lexiva®	1400 mg twice daily	Same as above	Tablets 700 mg
Indinavir	Crixivan®	800 mg every 8 hours	Protease inhibitor	Capsule 100 mg, 200 mg, 333 mg, 400 mg
Lopinavir/Ritonavir	Kaletra®	Lopinavir 800 mg/Ritonavir 200 mg once daily or Lopinavir 400 mg/ritonavir 100 mg twice daily	Same as above	Tablet Lopinavir 100 mg / Ritonavir 25 mg or Lopinavir 200 mg/ Ritonavir 50 mg
Nelfinavir	Viracept®	Adults 750 mg 3 times daily or 1250 mg twice daily	Same as above	Tablets 250 mg, 625 mg
Ritonavir	Norvir®	600 mg twice daily	Same as above	Capsule 100 mg, Solution 80 mg/ml
Saquinavir	Invirase®	Adults 1000 mg twice daily	Same as above	Tablet 500 mg, Capsule 200 mg
Tipranavir	Aptivus®	500 mg twice daily with a high fat meal; Must give with ritonavir 200 mg twice daily	Same as above	Capsules 250 mg

CHAPTER 24

ANTIFUNGALS

Disrupt Cell Membrane			Disrupt Cell Wall Synthesis- Echinocandins:	Stop Fungal Reproduction	
Inhibit Cell Membrane Synthesis		Cause cell membrane permeability:	caspofungin micafungin anidulafungin	Inhibit Nucleic Acid Synthesis (stop DNA synthesis):	Inhibit Microtubules:
Inhibit Synthesis of Lanosterol, a precursor to ergosterol	Inhibit Ergosterol Synthesis	amphotericin nystatin		flucytosine: inhibits thymidylate synthase, thus preventing DNA synthesis	griseofulvin
terbinafine naftine butenafine	ketoconazole fluconazole itraconazole voriconazole posaconazole				

Anti-fungal drugs work by three main mechanisms: 1) disrupting the cell membrane, 2) disrupting the cell wall, and 3) stopping fungal reproduction. The cell membrane can be disrupted by: 1) preventing the synthesis of ergosterol, a building block of fungal cell membranes or 2) physically altering the membrane's structure, causing holes to form, through which cellular contents leak out, lysing the cell. The cell wall (the outer most part) can be disrupted by preventing the synthesis of beta-(1,3)-D-glucan- a key building block of fungal cell walls. Without beta-(1,3)-D-glucan, the cell wall is unable to prevent excess water from flowing in and killing the cell. Finally, fungi can be stopped from reproducing by either inhibiting the synthesis of DNA building blocks, or by inhibiting microtubules from forming the mitotic spindle (a key step to separating DNA in fungal reproduction).

Ergosterol depends on the enzymes squalene epoxidase and 14-alpha-sterol demethylase for its production. Squalene epoxidase converts squalene to lanosterol. 14-alpha-sterol demethylase converts lanosterol to ergosterol. Without the production of ergoster-

ol, fungi cannot grow. Squalene epoxidase is inhibited by terbinafine, naftine, and butenafine. 14-alpha-sterol demethylase is inhibited by ketoconazole, fluconazole, itraconazole, voriconazole, and posaconazole. These drugs are usually bacteriostatic.

INHIBITING LANOSTEROL PRODUCTION

Squalene epoxidase inhibitors inhibit squalene epoxidase from converting squalene into lanosterol. These inhibitors include terbinafine, butenafine, and naftifine. Lanosterol is later converted to ergosterol by 14-alpha-sterol demethylase.

Terbinafine is approved to treat onychomycosis of toenails or fingernails caused by dermatophytes such as tinea unguium. To treat fingernail onychomycosis, patients take one 250mg tablet once daily for 6 weeks. To treat toenail onychomycosis, patients take one 250 mg tablet once daily for 12 weeks. Terbinafine causes headache, diarrhea, rash, dyspepsia, liver enzyme abnormalities, pruritus, taste disturbances, nausea, abdominal pain, and flatulence. More serious adverse effects include liver failure; check serum transaminases before starting therapy and check periodically thereafter.

INHIBITING ERGOSTEROL PRODUCTION

These drugs prevent the conversion of lanosterol to ergosterol by 14-alpha-sterol demethylase. 14-alpha-sterol demethylase inhibitors are structurally divided into the imidazole class and triazole class. Despite their structural differences, they both have the same mechanism of action. The triazoles include fluconazole, posaconazole, terconazole, and voriconazole. The imidazoles include ketoconazole, clotrimazole, miconazole, and econazole.

Ketoconazole is indicated to treat tinea versicolor caused by or presumed caused by *Pityrosporum orbiculare*. The affected area should be dampened before applying ketoconazole shampoo; it should be applied with a sufficient margin surrounding the affected area and left in place for 5 minutes, and then washed off. It is also used for tinea capitis, tinea corporis, and tinea cruris.

Fluconazole, a triazole anti-fungal, is indicated to treat vaginal candidiasis caused by *Candida*; oropharyngeal and esophageal candidiasis; and cryptococcal meningitis. Fluconazole is fungistatic.

It is available as an oral tablet, powder for oral suspension, and as an intravenous preparation. Fluconazole is over 90% absorbed after oral administration. Food does not affect its absorption. Fluconazole readily distributes to the CNS, saliva, sputum, vaginal tissue, and vaginal fluid. Most of the drug is excreted unchanged in the urine.

Fluconazole significantly increases the prothrombin time of warfarin. Fluconazole increases the plasma concentration of many drugs including cyclosporine, phenytoin, warfarin, zidovudine, and glipizide.

INHIBITORS OF CELL WALL SYNTHESIS

Fungal cell walls are, in part, made of beta-(1,3)-D-glucan. Fungal cell wall inhibitors, called echinocandins, inhibit the synthesis of beta-(1,3)-D-glucan. Without beta-(1,3)-D-glucan, excess water flows into the fungal cell, lysing it. Echinocandins include caspofungin, micafungin, and anidulafungin.

Caspofungin is indicated to treat presumed fungal infections in febrile, neutropenic patients; candidemia; esophageal candidiasis; and invasive aspergillosis in patients with infections that cannot be treated by amphotericin B, lipid formulations of amphotericin B, or itraconazole. Caspofungin is administered by slow intravenous infusion over one hour. For adults, on day one administer a 70 mg loading dose; on subsequent days administer 50 mg once daily for all indications (esophageal candidiasis does not require a loading dose). For adult patients on rifampin, use 70 mg once daily. Adverse reactions include diarrhea, pyrexia, increased ALT/AST levels, increased blood alkaline phosphatase levels, and decreased blood potassium levels. Cyclosporine substantially increases caspofungin's levels. P-glycoprotein does not affect caspofungin.

Anidulafungin is approved to treat candidemia and other forms of *Candida* infections and esophageal candidiasis. For candidemia and other forms of *Candida* infections, administer a 200 mg loading dose on day one, then 100 mg daily, continue for at least 14 days after the last positive culture. For esophageal candidiasis, administer a 100 mg loading dose on day one, followed by 50 mg daily for at least 14 days and at least 7 days after symptoms resolve. Do infuse faster than 1.1 mg/minute. Adverse reactions based on dosing for candidemia and other forms of *Candida* infections include diarrhea, nausea, vomiting, pyrexia, insomnia, and hypokalemia. Adverse reactions based on dosing for esophageal infections, include diarrhea, pyrexia, anemia, headache, vomiting, nausea, and dyspepsia.

Anidulafungin and cyclosporine do not affect each other's metabolism. Anidulafungin and tacrolimus do not significantly affect each other's metabolism. Rifampin does not alter the metabolism of anidulafungin. Anidulafungin and voriconazole do not significantly alter each other's metabolism.

Micafungin is approved to treat Candidemia, Acute Disseminated Candidiasis, *Candida* Peritonitis and Abscesses; esophageal candidiasis; and prophylaxis of Candida Infections in patients undergoing Hematopoietic Stem Cell Transplantation. For Candidemia, Acute Disseminated Candidiasis, *Candida* Peritonitis and Abscesses administer 100 mg once daily. For esophageal candidiasis, administer 150 mg once daily. For prophylaxis of *Candida* infections, administer 50 mg once daily. The dose should be infused over one hour.

Adverse reactions include diarrhea, nausea, vomiting, pyrexia, hypokalemia, thrombocytopenia, and headache. Anaphylaxis and anaphylactoid reactions have happened. Further, abnormalities in liver function tests, hepatic impairment, hepatitis, and hepatic failure have been observed with micafungin's use. Isolated occurrences of renal impairment or acute renal failure have happened.

Micafungin pharmacokinetics are not affected by amphotericin B, mycophenolate mofetil, cyclosporine, tacrolimus, prednisolone, sirolimus, nifedipine, fluconazole, itraconazole, voriconazole, ritonavir, and rifampin. Micafungin is not a substrate of P-glycoprotein.

DISRUPT CELL MEMBRANE PERMEABILITY

As with all types of cells, fungal cells must maintain a strong barrier around their intracellular contents (DNA, protein, intracellular ions etc.) to survive. Further, this barrier must prevent excess water from entering the cell. Amphotericin B and nystatin, both polyenes, bind with ergosterol, creating openings in the cell membrane, allowing intracellular ions (sodium, potassium, chloride, and hydrogen) to leave the cell, ultimately causing cell death. Their chemical structures, hydrophobic on one side and hydrophilic on the other side, allow these drugs to easily slide into the cell membrane, bind with ergosterol, and create openings for intracellular ions to exit the cell.

Amphotericin treats cryptococcal meningitis, *Aspergillus*, *Candida* species, *Cryptococcus* species, and visceral leishmaniasis. Intrathecal administration is necessary to achieve sufficient concentrations in the cerebrospinal fluid. Amphotericin can be fungicidal or fungistatic depending on its ability to infiltrate the cell membrane.

Amphotericin's nickname is "ampho-terrible" because of its severe side-effects. Because of these side-effects, amphotericin has been formulated in several different liposomal formulations, attempting to reduce its severe adverse-effects. These formulations include Amphotec®, Abelcet®, and AmBisome®.

Renal toxicity is a severe and common adverse effect of amphotericin. Amphotericin B also causes anemia.

Nystatin is used for topical skin infections, vaginal infections, and oral infections, especially in infants.

INHIBIT NUCLEIC ACID SYNTHESIS

Fungal cells need to produce DNA to reproduce. Thymidylate synthase is one of several important enzymes involved in producing DNA precursors. Flucytosine inhibits thymidylate synthase from producing deoxythymidylate- a necessary precursor to DNA production. Flucytosine also inhibits protein synthesis because it's similarity to cytosine causes it to be incorrectly added into RNA, making the RNA unreadable by ribosomes.

Flucytosine is approved to treat serious infections caused by susceptible strains of *Candida* and/or *Cryptococcus*. For systemic infections of candidiasis or cryptococcosis, flucytosine should be combined with amphotericin B.

Flucytosine has a black box warning of using it in patients with impaired renal function. Because flucytosine is mainly excreted by the kidneys, use it with extreme caution in patients with impaired renal function, as adverse blood levels may develop. Adjust the dose as necessary to prevent adverse accumulation of the drug. Check kidney function before starting therapy. Flucytosine may cause hypokalemia; check potassium blood levels before starting. Drugs interfering with kidney functioning may precipitously increase blood levels of flucytosine.

Several cardiac problems have occurred in patients using flucytosine, including cardiac arrest, myocardial toxicity, and ventricular dysfunction. Respiratory problems occurring in patients taking flucytosine include respiratory arrest, chest pain, and dyspnea. Myriad other adverse reactions have occurred in patients using flucytosine.

INHIBIT MICROTUBULES

Normally, microtubules function together to form a mitotic spindle. The mitotic spindle is a physical structure that separates DNA into two new cells after reproduction. Microtubules are formed from the combination of smaller pieces called "tubulin." Tubulin molecules join together to form microtubules. Griseofulvin physically binds with tubulin, consequently preventing the formation of the mitotic spindle, thus preventing cells from reproducing.

Griseofulvin treats dermatophytes of the hair, skin, and nails, including *Microsporum*, *Trichophyton*, and *Epidermophyton*. These infections include athlete's foot (tinea pedis), ring worm, jock itch (tinea cruris), scalp infections, and fingernail infections (tinea un-guium, onychomycosis). Griseofulvin is administered orally to treat these infections; it is not topically ad-ministered. Griseofulvin is usually reserved for severe infections that do not respond well to topical drugs such as nystatin.

Griseofulvin is generally well tolerated. It can cause headache, upset stomach, vomiting, and dizzi-ness.

Griseofulvin induces CYP450 enzymes. Of importance, it may decrease warfarin's levels, decreasing its effectiveness.

Anti-fungal Drugs: Polyenes Disrupt Cell Membrane

Generic Name/ Brand Name	Clinical Use	Dose	Mechanism of Action	Dosage Form
Amphotericin B Amphotec®	Systemic fungal infections, Asper-gillosis, crypto-coccosis	3-4 mg/kg/day IV	Binds to er-gosterol in the cell membrane causing cell death	Powder for reconstitution for injection
Nystatin Mycostatin® Nystop®	Oral Candidiasis, skin infections	For oral candidiasis for infants 100,000 units to each side of mouth 4 times daily; vaginal infections 1 tablet vaginally at bedtime for 14 days	Same as above	Oral Suspen-sion

Anti-fungal Drugs: Blocking Ergosterol Synthesis

Generic Name/ Brand Name	Clinical Use	Dose	Mechanism of Action	Dosage Form
Imidazoles				
Clotrimazole Lotrimin®	Skin infections	Adult oral fungal infection one 10 mg troche dissolved in mouth 5 times/day for 14 days	Inhibits ergosterol syn-thesis	Oral Troche 10 mg (Mycelex), cream 1%, cream vaginal 2%, solution 1%
Ketoconazole Nizoral®	Skin and scalp infections caused by *Pityrosporum orbiculare*	Adult fungal infections 200 mg-400 mg/day upto 6 months depending on infection	Same as above	Tablet 200 mg, Cream 2%, Sham-poo 1%
Miconazole Monistat®	Vaginal candi-diasis	1 suppository vaginally at bedtime for 7 nights. Ath-lete's foot apply twice daily for 14 days	Same as above	Many dosage forms are available under different names. Monistat 7 Combi-nation Pack
Triazoles				
Fluconazole Diflucan®	Vaginal infec-tions, some lung infections	150 mg tablet one time orally for vaginal yeast infection	Same as above	Tablets, Suspen-sion, IV

Anti-fungal Drugs: Blocking Ergosterol Synthesis

Generic Name/ Brand Name	Clinical Use	Dose	Mechanism of Action	Dosage Form
Voriconazole Vfend®	Invasive aspergillosis, candidemia, esophageal candidiasis, *Scedosporium apiospermum*, *Fusarium spp*.	People 12 and older 100 mg - 300 mg every 12 hours	Same as above	Tablet 50 mg, 200 mg; Powder for oral suspension 200 mg/5ml

Allylamines - Inhibiting lanosterol production

Terbinafine / Naftifine / and Butenafine	Nail infections caused by tinea unguium, onychomycosis	Adults athletes foot 250 mg once daily; Cream apply twice daily for 1 week	Inhibits production of lanosterol, which is a precursor to ergosterol	Terbinafine Tablets 250 mg, Cream 1%, Solution 1%; Butenafine 1% cream; and Naftifine 1% and 2% cream

Anti-fungal Drugs: Inhibiting Replication

Generic Name/ Brand Name	Clinical Use	Dose	Mechanism of Action	Dosage Form
Flucytosine Ancobon®	Systemic *Candida*, *Cryptococcus*	50-150 mg/kg/day in divided doses every 6 hours for several weeks depending on infection	Inhibits DNA synthesis, thus inhibiting cell replication	Capsule 250 mg, 500 mg
Griseofulvin Grifulvin V® Gris-PEG®	Skin, hair, nail infections from *Trichophyton*, *Epidermophyton*, *Microsporum*	Griseofulvin Microsize tablets 500 mg -1000mg daily in single or divided doses; Griseofulvin Ultramicrosize 375mg/day in single or divided doses	Inhibits fungal replication by inhibiting the process of separating DNA: mitosis	Grifulvin V Microsize 500 mg; Gris-PEG Ultramicrosize 125 mg, 250 mg, Suspension 125 mg/5ml

CHAPTER 25

ANTICANCER DRUGS

Anticancer drugs are divided into multiple classes. These classes include alkylating drugs, antimetabolites, natural products (vinca alkaloids, antibiotics, etc.), tyrosine kinase inhibitors, and monoclonal antibodies. Older anticancer drugs damage DNA, prevent the production of DNA building blocks, or inhibit DNA polymerase, among other mechanisms of action. Newer anticancer drugs (monoclonal antibodies and tyrosine kinase inhibitors) block growth signals and assist the immune system with lysing cancerous cells.

Anticancer drugs work at various stages of the cell cycle. The cell cycle consists of four stages which are the G_1, S, G_2, and M phases. During the G_1 phase, the cell undergoes normal growth. Cells may or may not enter a G_0 phase after G_1; in G_0 cells stop dividing. DNA replication occurs during the S phase. After the S phase, cells enter the G_2 phase. During the G_2 phase cells produce microtubules, which are structures used to separate replicated DNA. The M phase is when cells divide into two new cells. The M phase is subdivided into prophase, metaphase, anaphase, and telophase. The cell cycle is often depicted as a wheel. Each step of the cell cycle lasts a different length of time. G_1 is the longest phase, followed by the S phase, G_2 phase, and M phase in decreasing order. Drugs that work during the S phase have a longer time to act than the drugs affecting the G_2 phase or M phase.

ALKYLATING AGENTS

Alkylating agents physically attach to DNA, rendering DNA incapable of functioning properly. The various subgroups of alkylating drugs all work through the same general principle that a positively charged carbon atom (carbonium ion) covalently binds with the N7 nitrogen or O6 oxygen atom in guanine (a DNA base); these atoms have a pair of free electrons, which readily bind with carbonium ions; covalent bonds can also form with the DNA phosphate backbone. Most alkylating agents form covalent bonds with both strands of DNA (called cross-linking). Cross-linked DNA may not be able to be replicated, which often leads to cell death through apoptosis, which is preprogrammed cell death. Some cancer cells are able to survive even with alkylated DNA by excising alkylated DNA, a mecha-

nism of drug resistance. Other mechanisms of resistance include decreased cellular uptake of cancer agents and increased synthesis of biochemicals that bind with alkylating agents.

Alkylating agents are classified according to their physical structures. Alkylating agents include the nitrosoureas, nitrogen mustards, triazenes, and other drugs. Most alkylating agents have to be activated to their final reactive form that has a carbonium ion.

The nitrogen mustards include bendamustine chlorambucil, mechlorethamine, cyclophosphamide, ifosfamide, and melphalan. Nitrogen mustards agents affect rapidly growing cancer cells and normal healthy cells, such as blood cells. The nitrogen mustards are notable for their myelosuppressive property; blood cell counts should be monitored. They treat a range of cancers including leukemia, (see chart).

The nitrosoureas include carmustine and lomustine. Carmustine and lomustine treat brain cancers because they are able to cross the blood brain barrier, in contrast to many other agents. Carmustine has a black box warning for pulmonary toxicity. The risk increases substantially as the total cumulative dose exceeds 1400 mg/m². Lomustine causes bone marrow toxicity, which depends on the total dose that a patient has received.

The triazenes include dacarbazine. Dacarbazine requires CYP450 activation to its active metabolite (MTIC). Dacarbazine treats malignant melanoma and Hodgkin's Disease. Dacarbazine causes myelosuppression. Temozolomide, another triazene, is also metabolized to MTIC.

SIDE-EFFECTS

Alkylating agents affect rapidly growing cells, which include gastrointestinal cells, blood cells, hair cells, and cells inside the mouth. Alkylating agents cause bone marrow suppression or myelosuppression (a decreased amount of red blood cells, white blood cells, and platelets). Infections are a common result of chemotherapeutic drugs, including alkylating drugs. Hair loss (alopecia), oral ulcers, and damage to the gastrointestinal tract result from alkylating agents. These agents can also cause secondary malignancies.

Cyclophosphamide is particularly harmful to

the bladder; however the drug mesna can negate the harmful actions against the bladder.

When given in large cumulative doses, carmustine and lomustine have caused renal failure. Pulmonary fibrosis can occur years after carmustine use. Leukemia may result from carmustine or lomustine. Chlorambucil causes infertility. It is also teratogenic.

Infusion reactions can occur with bendamustine; severe reactions necessitate discontinuing it. For Grade 1 or 2 reactions, patients can be pre-treated with antihistamines, corticosteroids, and acetaminophen.

DRUG INTERACTIONS

Cimetidine increases the incidence of carmustine induced leukopenia and neutropenia. Bendamustine is metabolized by CYP1A2; bendamustine has active metabolites. CYP1A2 inducers may increase levels of bendamustine's active metabolites, and the converse of inhibitors of CYP1A2. Bendamustine itself does not cause interactions through the CYP system.

PLATINUM ANALOGS

Platinum analogs treat bladder, testicular, ovarian, colon cancer, esophagus, head, lung, and neck cancers. Cisplatin, oxaliplatin, and carboplatin work in a similar manner to alkylating drugs. Inside cells, platinum analogs react with water to create a new molecule that has a positively charged platinum atom. This positively charged platinum atom reacts with the free electrons of nitrogen (N-7 nitrogen) in a guanine DNA base pair, resulting in platinum and guanine bonded together. This platinum atom can then bind with another nitrogen atom either on the same DNA strand (intra-strand cross-link) or bind with nitrogen in a guanine base pair on the corresponding DNA strand (inter-strand cross-linking). Decreased uptake of platinum analogs is a mechanism of resistance used by some cancer cells.

SIDE-EFFECTS

Cisplatin and oxaliplatin both cause peripheral neuropathy. Carboplatin can cause neurotoxicity. All can cause myelosuppression, pulmonary fibrosis, and leukemia. Myelosuppression is the dose-limiting side-effect of carboplatin.

ANTIMETABOLITES

Antimetabolites include:
- Anti-folates (methotrexate, etc.),
- Pyrimidine analogs (fluorouracil, etc.), and
- Purine analogs (mercaptopurine, etc.).

ANTI-FOLATES

Anti-folates block the production of DNA base pairs. DNA base pair construction depends on the availability of methyl groups, which are needed to produce DNA base pairs. Methotrexate, pemetrexed, and pralatrexate inhibit the enzyme dihydrofolate reductase from converting dihydrofolate to tetrahydrofolate, the source of methyl groups used to construct DNA base pairs. Methotrexate, pemetrexed, and pralatrexate all inhibit the conversion of dihydrofolates to tetrahydrofolates. These drugs enter cells through the reduced folate transporter (SLC19A1 transporter).

Methotrexate treats acute lymphoblastic leukemia (ALL) in children. Methotrexate treats meningeal leukemia, breast cancer, head and neck cancers, cutaneous T-Cell lymphoma, lung cancer, and advanced non-Hodgkin's lymphomas. Pemetrexed treats non-squamous non-small cell lung cancer and mesothelioma. Pralatrexate treats relapsed or refractory peripheral T-cell lymphoma (PTCL).

SIDE-EFFECTS

Methotrexate and its analogs all cause myelosuppression and gastrointestinal problems. Leucovorin (folinic acid) treats hematological crisis resulting from myelosuppression. Leucovorin, a reduced folate, allows cells to produce DNA. Methotrexate causes liver problems. Liver biopsies should be conducted when a total cumulative dose of 1-1.5 grams is reached.

DRUG INTERACTIONS

Methotrexate highly binds to plasma proteins. Consequently, administering methotrexate with other drugs that highly bind to plasma protein displaces methotrexate from plasma proteins, increasing the amount of free methotrexate that can cause myelosuppression.

PYRIMIDINE ANALOGS

Pyrimidine analogs include capecitabine, fluorouracil, gemcitabine, azacytidine, and cytarabine. Despite their structural similarities, pyrimidine analogs do not all have the same mechanism of action.

Fluorouracil, a prodrug, inhibits the enzyme thymidylate synthase, blocking production of the nucleotide thymidine, a necessary building block of DNA. Fluorouracil is approved to treat breast, colon, rectum, pancreas, and stomach cancers. Capecitabine is a prodrug of fluorouracil. Some cancer cells resist fluorouracil.

Cytarabine inhibits DNA polymerase from adding DNA base pairs to a growing strand of DNA. Cytarabine becomes biologically active after the addition of a monophosphate group. Cytarabine is incorrectly added to a growing DNA strand which prevents DNA polymerase from adding more DNA base pairs. Inhibition of DNA polymerase prevents DNA replication and repairing of DNA. This inhibition of replication, or, second, blocking of DNA repair, usually leads to apoptosis. Cytarabine works during the "S" phase of the cell cycle. Cytarabine has a black box warning indicating that it causes myelosuppression (leukopenia, thrombocytopenia, and anemia). Cytarabine carries a black box warning for chemical arachnoiditis (nausea, vomiting, headache, and/or fever), which occurs commonly and may be fatal if not promptly treated. Both the incidence and severity of chemical arachnoiditis are reduced when DepoCyt® is administered with dexamethasone. Cytarabine may also cause neurotoxicity, the risk of which is amplified when administered with other CNS toxic drugs. Cytarabine is for intrathecal use only.

Cytarabine treats acute myeloid leukemia (AML), acute lymphocytic leukemia (ALL), chronic myelocytic leukemia (CML), and meningeal leukemia.

Gemcitabine is approved to treat metastatic breast cancer, inoperable locally advanced or metastatic non-small cell lung cancer (NSCLC), locally advanced or metastatic pancreatic cancer, or relapsed ovarian cancer. Gemcitabine, after the necessary phosphorylation, inhibits both ribonucleotide reductase and DNA polymerase; two enzymes needed to produce DNA. After being incorrectly added to a growing DNA strand, gemcitabine inhibits DNA polymerase, causing DNA strand termination, leading to apoptosis. It commonly causes myelosuppression.

PURINE ANALOGS

Purine analogs include fludarabine, cladribine, clofarabine, mercaptopurine, and thioguanine. Thioguanine, after phosphorylation, inhibits the conversion of inosine-5'-monophosphate to guanine. It is also incorporated into a growing strand of DNA, causing DNA strand breaks and apoptosis. Thioguanine is approved to treat acute myelogenous (non-lymphocytic) leukemia (AML). Thioguanine causes myelosuppression and liver toxicity.

Mercaptopurine inhibits the production of adenine, a DNA base. Mercaptopurine inhibits the conversion of inosine-5'-monophosphate to adenine or guanine, thus inhibiting DNA synthesis. Fatal hepatic necrosis has occurred with mercaptopurine. Leukopenia, thrombocytopenia, and anemia are common side-effects. It is approved as a component of maintenance therapy for acute lymphoblastic leukemia (ALL).

Fludarabine (Fludara®) is incorporated into DNA, which then stops elongation of that strand. It also inhibits DNA polymerase, DNA primase, and DNA ligase I. It is also incorrectly incorporated into RNA strands, thus inhibiting RNA functioning. It is approved to treat progressive or refractory B-cell chronic lymphocytic leukemia (CLL). Fludarabine, at higher than recommended doses, may cause neurological toxicity including delayed blindness, coma, and death. At standard doses, it has also caused neurotoxicity including agitation, coma, confusion, and seizure.

NATURAL PRODUCTS

Natural products include antibiotics (doxorubicin, bleomycin), camptothecins, epipodophyllotoxins (etoposide), taxanes (paclitaxel), and vinca alkaloids.

VINCA ALKALOIDS

The vinca alkaloids include vinblastine, vincristine, and vinorelbine. The vinca alkaloids inhibit the formation of microtubules. Specifically, vinca alkaloids bind with beta-tubulin, thus preventing beta-tubulin from binding with alpha-tubulin, which in turn prevents the formation of microtubules. Without microtubules, cells cannot divide properly, apoptosis ensues. Vinblastine is approved to treat testicular cancer, breast cancer, mycosis fungoides, Kaposi's Sarcoma, histiocytosis, and choriocarcinoma. Vinblastine may cause death if given intrathecally.

Vincristine is approved to treat acute lympho-cytic leukemia (ALL), Hodgkin's lymphoma, non-Hodgkin's lymphoma, Wilm's tumor, neuroblastoma, and rhabdomyosarcoma. Never administer vincristine intrathecally; it will cause severe neurological damage and/or death. Additionally, vincristine, if extravasation occurs, can cause cellulitis and phlebitis. Vincristine, of all the vinca alkaloids, causes the least amount of myelosuppression.

Vinorelbine is approved to treat non-small cell lung cancer. Vinorelbine is fatal if administered intra-thecally. Vinorelbine is metabolized by CYP3A subfam-ily.

TAXANES

Paclitaxel and docetaxel compose the taxane class of drugs. The taxanes, in contrast to the vinca al-kaloids, promote the assembly of microtubules by bind-ing with beta-tubulin, but also prevent the disassembly of microtubules once they are formed, thus preventing cells from replicating. Apoptosis follows after stopping microtubule disassembly. Paclitaxel is approved to treat breast cancer, non-small cell lung cancer, ovarian cancer, and AIDS-related Kaposi's Sarcoma. It has a black box warning of bone marrow suppression and hypersensitivity reactions. Administer dexamethasone, diphenhydramine, and cimetidine as pretreatment for hypersensitivity reactions. Nab-paclitaxel, a nano-par-ticle solution of paclitaxel bound to albumin, does not cause the same hypersensitivity reaction. However, both cause peripheral neuropathy.

Docetaxel is approved to treat breast cancer, lo-cally-advanced or metastatic non-small cell lung cancer, hormone refractory metastatic prostate cancer, ad-vanced gastric adenocarcinoma, and locally-advanced squamous cell head and neck cancer.

EPIPODOPHYLLOTOXINS

Etoposide and teniposide both bind with topoisomerase II while topoisomerase II is bound to DNA. These drugs prevent topoisomerase II from resealing the breaks in DNA strands that occur during DNA replication. Preventing the resealing of breaks in DNA strands eventually causes cell death. Etoposide is approved to treat refractory testicular tumors and small cell lung cancer. Myelosuppression is the dose-limiting side-effect associated with etoposide. Anaphylactic reactions have occurred.

Teniposide (VM-26), in combination with oth-er anticancer drugs, is approved for induction therapy for refractory childhood acute lymphoblastic leukemia. A common side-effect of teniposide is myelosuppres-sion; patients should be monitored for this during and after therapy. Teniposide can cause hypersensitivity reactions. If necessary, patients should be treated with antihistamines, corticosteroids, epinephrine, intrave-nous fluids, and other necessary steps.

CAMPTOTHECINS

Irinotecan and topotecan both inhibit to-poisomerase I. Topoisomerase I binds with DNA and then unwinds DNA by cleaving a single strand of DNA, allowing the DNA's physical shape to be changed so it can be replicated. Topoisomerase I then rejoins the cleaved strands of DNA. Irinotecan and topotecan both bind to topoisomerase I while it is bound to DNA. The binding of irinotecan or topotecan to the DNA-to-poisomerase complex prevents topoisomerase I from rejoining the cleaved strands of DNA. Ultimately, this causes a double-strand break leading to cell death.

Irinotecan is approved to treat metastatic carci-noma of the colon or rectum. It has a black box warn-ing for severe diarrhea (possibly fatal), severe myelo-suppression (death from sepsis), and cases of interstitial pulmonary disease causing death have occurred. Before IV infusion, patients should receive dexamethasone and a 5-HT$_3$ antagonist (ondansetron). The liver metaboliz-es it to its active metabolite SN-38.

Topotecan is approved to treat small cell lung cancer sensitive disease after failure of first line chemo-therapy. It has a black box warning for neutropenia. Leukopenia is the dose-limiting side-effect if topotecan. After IV infusion, about 50% of topotecan is excreted unchanged in the urine.

ANTIBIOTIC ANTICANCER DRUGS

The antibiotics include dactinomycin, doxoru-bicin, daunorubicin, idarubicin and epirubicin.

Antibiotic-anticancer drugs intercalate between DNA base pairs. This intercalation interferes with to-poisomerase II, eventually leading to breaks in the DNA which in turn cause apoptosis. Intercalation means the drug enters DNA between two DNA base pairs (roughly analogous to adding a card between two cards in a deck of cards). Intercalated drugs physically hinder RNA polymerase from functioning.

Dactinomycin, used in combination with other drugs, is approved to treat Wilms' tumor, childhood rhabdomyosarcoma, Ewing's sarcoma, and metastatic non-seminomatous testicular cancer.

Epirubicin treats primary breast cancer. Idarubicin is approved to treat acute myeloid leukemia (AML) in adults. Daunorubicin treats acute lymphocytic leukemia (ALL) and acute myeloid leukemia (AML). Doxorubicin treats acute lymphoblastic leukemia, acute myeloblastic leukemia, and many other disorders.

All of these agents can cause myocardial toxicity. Doxorubicin, idarubicin, and epirubicin all can cause severe myelosuppression.

EGFR INHIBITORS: MONOCLONAL ANTIBODIES

Epidermal growth factor (EGF) regulates the growth and differentiation of epithelial cells. Normal cells receive the appropriate amount of stimulation from EGF so they do not over grow. In contrast, EGF excessively stimulates some cells, thus causing them to become cancerous.

Epidermal growth factor binds to the Epidermal Growth Factor Receptor (EGFR). EGFR has an intracellular domain and an extracellular domain. EGF binds with the extracellular domain, activating intracellular kinases that signal the cell nucleus to replicate the cell. EGFR's intracellular domain is a tyrosine kinase - an enzyme that phosphorylates tyrosine on messenger-proteins. Drugs can either block the extracellular domain or intracellular domain.

Cetuximab and panitumumab, two monoclonal antibodies, block the extracellular domain of EGFR, thus blocking epidermal growth factor from binding to EGFR, thus reducing abnormal cell growth. Cetuximab, in vitro, can activate antibody-dependent cellular cytotoxicity, which prompts the immune system to lyse cancerous cells. Cetuximab is approved as mono-therapy for metastatic colon cancer. Panitumumab is approved to treat metastatic colorectal cancer.

EGFR TYROSINE KINASE INHIBITORS

Erlotinib is approved to treat metastatic pancreatic cancer and non-small cell lung cancer. Gefitinib is approved to treat patients with locally advanced or metastatic non-small cell lung cancer.

Erlotinib and gefitinib are tyrosine kinase inhibitors. They block the intracellular domain of EGFR, thus preventing EGFR from transmitting growth signals to the nucleus of the cell. Specifically, they stop the intracellular domain of EGFR from phosphorylating a tyrosine amino-acid of a messenger-protein, a messenger that propagates growth signals to the cell nucleus.

HER-2 INHIBITORS

Trastuzumab treats HER2 positive breast cancer. As a monoclonal antibody, it binds to and blocks the extracellular domain of human epidermal growth factor receptor-2 protein (HER-2). This prevents the tyrosine kinase part of the receptor (inside the cell) from phosphorylating other proteins that act as second messengers, thus stopping growth signals from reaching the cell nucleus.

Lapatinib also blocks the growth signal pathway of HER2, but it works on the inside of the cancer cell as opposed to the outside. It blocks tyrosine kinase from phosphorylating secondary messenger proteins.

Lapatinib with capecitabine treats advanced or metastatic breast cancer. It is also approved, for use with letrozole, to treat post-menopausal women who have hormone receptor positive metastatic breast. Lapatinib is associated with hepatotoxicity and interstitial lung disease. It may cause severe diarrhea.

Lapatinib inhibits metabolism of drugs that are substrates of CYP3A4 and CYP2C8. Dose of midazolam may need to be lowered when administered with lapatinib. It also inhibits P-glycoprotein, substantially increasing exposure to digoxin.

BCR-ABL TYROSINE KINASE INHIBITORS

Dasatinib, imatinib, and nilotinib are tyrosine kinase inhibitors approved to treat chronic myeloid leukemia (CML). CML results from an abnormal tyrosine kinase called BCR-ABL.

All three are metabolized by CYP3A4; hence drugs that induce or inhibit CYP3A4 will affect blood levels of these drugs. As oral drugs, all three can cause nausea, however, dose-reduction is usually adequate to address this side-effect.

VASCULAR ENDOTHELIAL GROWTH FACTOR INHIBITORS

As fast growing cells, cancer cells need new blood vessels to supply nutrients for growth. Bevacizumab, a monoclonal antibody, blocks the growth of new blood vessels that cancer cells cause to form. Cancer cells depend on vascular endothelial growth factor (VEGF) to stimulate new blood vessel growth. Bevacizumab physically binds with VEGF, preventing VEGF from binding with its receptor, vascular endothelial growth factor receptor, which has three subtypes VEGFR-1 , VEGFR-2, and VEGFR-3 (all are receptor tyrosine kinases).

Bevacizumab is approved to treat metastatic colorectal cancer in combination with 5-fluorouracil and non-squamous non-small cell lung cancer, among other indications. It has black box warnings for gastrointestinal perforation, wound healing complications, and severe or fatal hemorrhage, including hemoptysis, central nervous system hemorrhage, epistaxis, and vaginal bleeding. Further, serious pulmonary hemorrhage has occurred in patients with non-small cell lung cancer. Bevacizumab may also cause stroke or myocardial infarction. It also causes hypertension, which usually must be treated.

As opposed to binding with VEGF itself, **sunitinib** and **sorafenib** block the vascular endothelial growth factor receptor, preventing growth signals from reaching cell nuclei.

Sorafenib inhibits VEGFR-1, VEGFR-2, and VEGFR-3, in addition to many other kinases. It is approved to treat un-resectable hepatocellular carcinoma and advanced renal cell carcinoma. It is usually dosed at 400 mg (two tablets) twice daily without food. Some patients, because of side-effects, require a dose reduction to 400 mg once daily or every other day.

Sunitinib inhibits VEGFR-2, PDGFR-beta, and KIT, in addition to many other kinases. It is approved to treat gastrointestinal stromal tumor, advanced renal cell carcinoma, and pancreatic neuroendocrine tumors. Sunitinib has caused both severe and fatal hepatotoxicity. Ketoconazole, a strong CYP3A4 inhibitor, substantially increases sunitinib levels.

HEMATOPOIETIC DRUGS

Anticancer drugs reduce immune system cells, red blood cells, and platelets, leading to infections, anemia, and bleeding. Hematopoietic drugs raise counts of white blood cells, red blood cells, and platelets. All of the hematopoietic drugs are proteins that must be administered by injection.

Erythropoietin and darbepoetin both increase the production of red blood cells by binding with erythropoietin receptors on progenitor cells, stimulating increased production of red blood cells. Darbepoetin is a structurally modified version of erythropoietin, providing it with a longer half-life. Both have black box warnings on their package inserts explaining that both shortened survival and/or increased the risk of tumor progression or recurrence in studies of patients with breast, non-small cell lung, head and neck, lymphoid, and cervical cancers. Further, both have black box warnings explaining that they cause myocardial infarction, stroke, venous thromboembolism, thrombosis of vascular access and tumor progression or recurrence.

Erythropoietin and darbepoetin are indicated to treat anemia caused by 1) chronic kidney disease (CKD) and 2) anemia in patients receiving myelosuppressive chemotherapy. Erythropoietin is also indicated to treat anemia caused by zidovudine therapy.

Sargramostim, filgrastim, and pegfilgrastim all promote the growth of white blood cells for patients receiving chemotherapy. Sargramostim binds with receptors on myeloid stem cells and progenitor cells causing myeloid stem cells and progenitor cells to differentiate into neutrophils. Filgrastim, and peg-filgrastim cause progenitor cells to differentiate into neutrophils. Peg-filgrastim is filgrastim with polyethylene glycol added, increasing the half-life of the drug. Filgrastim and pegfilgrastim have caused splenic rupture, sometimes fatal. Filgrastim and pegfilgrastim have also caused acute respiratory distress syndrome, resulting from excess neutrophils entering the lungs. Filgrastim and pegfilgrastim commonly cause bone pain; it can usually be treated with non-opioid drugs.

Some chemotherapy drugs decrease platelet counts. Oprelvekin stimulates the production of megakaryocytes and their maturation into platelets. It is indicated to prevent severe thrombocytopenia in adult patients who are at risk of thrombocytopenia after myelosuppressive chemotherapy for nonmyeloid malignancies. It is not indicated for patients receiving myeloablative chemotherapy; these patients experience a statistically significant increase in edema, conjunctival bleeding, hypotension, and tachycardia.

DNA Alkylating Agents			
Generic Name Brand Name	Indications	Warnings and Adverse Reactions	Mechanism of Action
Nitrogen Mustards - Non phase specific			
Bendamustine Treanda®	Chronic lymphocytic leukemia; Indolent B-cell non-Hodgkin's lymphoma	Myelosuppression, Tumor lysis syndrome, Severe skin reactions	Alkylates both strands of DNA (bifunctional), forming cross-links between DNA strands, which leads to cell death
Chlorambucil Leukeran®	Chronic lymphatic leukemia, lymphosarcoma, giant follicular lymphoma, Hodgkin's disease	Myelosuppression Hepatotoxicity Seizures Secondary malignancies Infertility	Same as above
Cyclophosphamide Cytoxan®	Hodgkin's and Non-Hodgkin's lymphoma	Alopecia Myelosuppression	Same as above
Ifosfamide Ifex®	Germ cell testicular cancer (third-line use)	Myelosuppression Neurotoxicity Renal failure	Same as above
Mechlorethamine Mustargen®	Palliative treatment of Hodgkin's disease (stages III and IV), lymphosarcoma, chronic myelocytic or chronic lymphocytic leukemia	Hyperuricemia Myelosuppression Decreased renal and kidney functioning	Same as above
Melphalan Alkeran®	Palliative treatment of multiple myeloma, palliation of non-resectable epithelial carcinoma of the ovary	Myelosuppression Secondary malignancies including leukemia	Same as above
Nitrosureas			
Carmustine BiCNU®	Brain tumors, multiple myeloma with prednisone, Hodgkin's disease, Non-Hodgkin's lymphomas	Delayed bone marrow suppression, Secondary malignancies including leukemia	Same as above

DNA Alkylating Agents			
Lomustine CeeNU®	Brain tumors, and Hodgkin's disease	Delayed bone marrow suppression Renal failure at high doses Kidney damage at low doses, Secondary malignancies including leukemia	Alkylates DNA and RNA, leading to cell death
Additional DNA Alkylating Agents			
Altretamine Hexalen®	Palliative treatment of ovarian cancer	Myelosuppression Neurotoxicity Anaphylaxis	Alkylates one DNA strand; Also degrades to toxic substances that kill the cancer cell
Busulfan Myleran®	Palliative treatment of chronic myelogenous leukemia	Bone marrow failure (pancytopenia)	Alkylates both strands of DNA (bifunctional), forming cross-links between DNA strands, disrupting DNA replication
Dacarbazine	Malignant melanoma, Hodgkin's Disease	Myelosuppression	Alkylates DNA
Temozolomide (Derivative of dacarbazine) Temodar®	Newly diagnosed glioblastoma multiforme, Refractory anaplastic astrocytoma	Myelosuppression Secondary malignancies Alopecia	Alkylates one strand of DNA, does not produce bifunctional cross-links.
Thiotepa	Superficial bladder cancer	Myelosuppression Alopecia	Same as above
Platinum Complexes			
Carboplatin Paraplatin®	Ovarian cancer	Myelosuppression (dose limiting) Anaphylaxis	Covalently bind with DNA, creating inter-strand and intra-strand cross-links, preventing DNA replication and transcription
Cisplatin Platinol®	Bladder, testicular, and ovarian cancer	Myelosuppression Renal toxicity	Same as above
Oxaliplatin Eloxatin®	Adjuvant treatment of stage III colon cancer, treatment of advanced colorectal cancer,	Pulmonary toxicity Neuropathy Hepatotoxicity	Same as above

Antimetabolites			
Generic Name Brand Name	Indications	Warnings and Adverse Reactions	Mechanism of Action
Methotrexate and derivatives			
Methotrexate	Gestational choriocarcinoma, chorioadenoma destruens, hydatidiform mole, acute lymphocytic leukemias, breast cancer, epidermoid cancers of the head and neck, cutaneous T-cell lymphoma, and lung cancer	Myelosuppression Hepatotoxicity Diarrhea Hemorrhagic enteritis	Prevents synthesis of reduced folates
Pemetrexed Alimta®	Non-squamous non-small cell lung cancer, mesothelioma	Myelosuppression Fatigue, nausea, anorexia	Same as above. Also inhibits thymidylate synthase
Pralatrexate Folotyn®	Treatment of relapsed or refractory peripheral T-cell lymphoma (PTCL)	Mucositis Thrombocytopenia Pyrexia Sepsis	Same as above
Purine Analogs			
Cladribine Leustatin®	Hairy cell leukemia	Anemia Neutropenia Thrombocytopenia	Incorporated into DNA, thus preventing replication.
Fludarabine Fludara®	B-cell chronic lymphocytic leukemia (CLL)	Pulmonary toxicity Coma Seizures Agitation	Inhibits DNA synthesis by 1) inhibiting DNA Polymerase, 2) inhibits ribonucleotide reductase, 3) inhibits DNA primase.
Mercaptopurine (6-MP) Purinethol®	Acute lymphoblastic leukemia (ALL)	Myelosuppression Hepatotoxicity Renal toxicity	Incorporated into a growing DNA strand or RNA strand, then prevents further growth of that strand, the next DNA base pair or RNA base pair cannot be attached
Pentostatin Nipent®	Hairy cell leukemia	CNS toxicity Renal toxicity Hepatotoxicity Pulmonary toxicity	Inhibits DNA synthesis by blocking ribonucleotide reductase
Thioguanine (6-TG) Tabloid®	Acute myelogenous leukemia	Liver toxicity Myelosuppression	Incorporated into DNA and RNA, thus preventing replication and prevents guanine synthesis

Antimetabolites			
Generic Name Brand Name	Indications	Warnings and Adverse Reactions	Mechanism of Action
Pyrimidine Analogs			
5-Fluorouracil (5-FU) Carac®, Efudex®	Fluorouracil (IV): palliative treatment of colon, rectum, breast, stomach, and pancreas carcinomas Carac®: multiple actinic or solar keratoses of the face and anterior scalp	Alopecia Stomatitis Leukopenia Thrombocytopenia Gastrointestinal hemorrhage	Prevents DNA production by blocking the methylation of deoxyuridylic acid, which prevents synthesis of thymidylic acid, thus preventing DNA synthesis
Capecitabine Xeloda®	Colorectal cancer, Metastatic breast cancer	Bleeding /death when administered with warfarin. Severe diarrhea Cardiotoxicity Neutropenia Thrombocytopenia	Prodrug of fluorouracil. Blocks the conversion of deoxyuridylic acid to thymidylic acid.
Cytarabine Depocyt®	Intrathecal treatment of lymphomatous meningitis	Chemical arachnoiditis (potentially fatal),	Inhibits DNA Polymerase preventing DNA synthesis and repair. Also incorporated into DNA which then prevents DNA elongation, leading to cell death
Gemcitabine Gemzar®	Ovarian cancer, metastatic breast cancer, non-small cell lung cancer, pancreatic cancer,	Myelosuppression Pulmonary toxicity Renal failure Nausea Vomiting Anemia	Inhibits DNA Polymerase and inhibits ribonucleotide reductase.

Microtubule Disruptors			
Generic Name Brand Name	Indications	Warnings and Adverse Reactions	Mechanism of Action
Docetaxel Taxotere®	Breast cancer, Non-small cell lung cancer	Anaphylaxis Myelosuppression Neuropathy	Promotes formation of microtubules, but then prevents their disassembly, stopping cell growth
Paclitaxel Taxol®	Breast cancer, non-small cell lung cancer, ovarian cancer	Anaphylaxis Myelosuppression Neuropathy	Same as above
Vinblastine	Hodgkin's and Non-Hodgkin's lymphoma, breast, head, lung, neck, and renal carcinomas	Myelosuppression	By binding to beta tubulin, vinblastine inhibits microtubule formation.
Vincristine Vincasar® PFS	Leukemias, Hodgkin's disease, non-Hodgkin's lymphoma.	Myelosuppression Peripheral neuropathy	Same as above

Microtubule Disruptors			
Generic Name Brand Name	Indications	Warnings and Adverse Reactions	Mechanism of Action
Vinorelbine Navelbine®	Non-small cell lung cancer	Granulocytopenia	Same as above

Antibiotic Anticancer Drugs			
Generic Name Brand Name	Indications	Warnings and Adverse Reactions	Mechanism of Action
Bleomycin Blenoxane®	Squamous cell carcinoma, Hodgkin's disease, non-Hodgkin's lymphoma, testicular carcinoma, malignant pleural effusion	Pulmonary fibrosis Pneumonitis	Binds to DNA causing single and double strand DNA breaks in G2 and mitosis.
Dactinomycin Cosmegen®	Wilms' tumor, childhood rhabdomyosarcoma, Ewing's sarcoma, and metastatic, non-seminomatous testicular cancer	Extravasation severely damages soft tissues. Myelosuppression Leukemia Alopecia	Inserts itself (intercalates) between DNA subunits, preventing proper DNA functioning
Doxorubicin Adriamycin®	Leukemias, lymphomas, multiple myeloma	Cardiotoxicity Myelosuppression Alopecia	Intercalates between DNA base pairs, which interferes with topoisomerase II, causing DNA strand breaks
Daunorubicin Hydrochloride (Cerubidine)	Acute lymphocytic leukemia (ALL) and acute nonlymphocytic leukemias (ANLL)	Myelosuppression Alopecia Cardiotoxicity	Same as above
Idarubicin Idamycin® PFS	Acute myeloid leukemia	Extravasation severely damages soft tissues. Myocardial toxicity Myelosuppression Reduce dose with decreased hepatic or renal function	Intercalates between DNA base pairs preventing replication
Epirubicin Ellence®	Adjuvant therapy for primary breast cancer	Extravasation severely damages soft tissues. Myelosuppression Cardiac toxicity Secondary acute myelogenous leukemia	Intercalates between DNA base pairs preventing replication or synthesis. Intercalation causes topoisomerase II to cleave DNA, resulting in cell death
Mitoxantrone Novantrone®	Advanced hormone refractory prostate cancer, acute non-lymphocytic leukemia	Extravasation severely damages soft tissues. Bone marrow suppression Neutropenia Cardiotoxicity Secondary acute myeloid leukemia	Intercalates between DNA base pairs, causing DNA strand breaks; inhibits topoisomerase II

Antibiotic Anticancer Drugs			
Generic Name Brand Name	Indications	Warnings and Adverse Reactions	Mechanism of Action
Mitomycin Mutamycin®	Adenocarcinoma of stomach or pancreas, bladder cancer, breast cancer, colorectal cancer	Bone marrow suppression	Intercalates between DNA base pairs preventing replication or synthesis

Monoclonal Antibodies			
Generic Name Brand Name	Indications	Warnings and Adverse Reactions	Mechanism of Action
Alemtuzumab Campath®	B-cell chronic lymphocytic leukemia (B-CLL)	Pancytopenia Infections Serious and possibly fatal infusion reactions.	Binds to the CD52 antigen on B lymphocytes, allowing immune cells to lyse leukemic B lymphocytes
Bevacizumab Avastin®	Metastatic colorectal cancer; non-squamous non-small cell lung cancer, glioblastoma, metastatic renal cell carcinoma	Gastrointestinal perforation, hemorrhage, complications for surgery and wound healing,	Binds with VEGF, preventing VEGF from binding with its receptors, preventing new blood vessel growth
Cetuximab Erbitux®	Squamous cell carcinoma of the head and neck, K-ras mutation-negative EGFR-expressing metastatic colorectal cancer	Infusion reactions Cardiopulmonary arrest Pulmonary toxicity Dermatologic toxicity Hypomagnesemia	Binds with the epidermal growth factor receptor (EGFR), preventing epidermal growth factor from binding with EGFR
Gemtuzumab Mylotarg®	CD33 positive acute myeloid leukemia (AML) in first relapse for patients 60 years and older and no other treatment is available	Myelosuppression Anaphylaxis Infusion reactions Pulmonary events Hepatotoxicity	As an antibody to the CD33 antigen, it binds to CD33, and is then brought into the cell, part of the drug breaks off and enters the cell nucleus and binds with DNA, causing DNA strand breaks, leading to cell death
Panitumumab Vectibix®	Metastatic colorectal cancer, not for patients with *KRAS* mutation-positive mCRC or when *KRAS* mCRC status is unknown	Dermatologic toxicity Infusion reactions Pulmonary fibrosis Electrolyte depletion Ocular toxicities	IgG2 monoclonal antibody, it binds with epidermal growth factor receptor, blocking EGF and other ligands, inhibiting growth of cancer cells.
Rituxamab Rituxan®	Non-Hodgkin's Lymphoma, Chronic Lymphocytic Leukemia, Rheumatoid arthritis, granulomatosis with polyangiitis (GPA), and microscopic polyangiitis	Bowel obstruction and perforation, Cardiac arrhythmias Tumor lysis syndrome Lymphopenia Neutropenia	Fab domain binds with CD20 antigen on B lymphocytes, then the Fc domain attracts immune cells to lyse B lymphocytes

Monoclonal Antibodies

Generic Name Brand Name	Indications	Warnings and Adverse Reactions	Mechanism of Action
Trastuzumab Herceptin®	Adjuvant breast cancer, metastatic breast cancer, metastatic gastric cancer	Infusion reactions Cardiomyopathy Pulmonary toxicity Neutropenia	IgG1 monoclonal antibody. Binds to extracellular domain of HER-2 receptor, causing antibody-dependent cellular cytotoxicity (Trastuzumab binds with cells that have the HER-2 receptor then attracts immune cells to lyse that cell, HER-2 is found on cancer cell.)

Topoisomerase Inhibitors

Generic Name Brand Name	Indications	Warnings and Adverse Reactions	Mechanism of Action
Etoposide Toposar®	Testicular cancer, Small cell lung cancer	Severe myelosuppression Anaphylaxis Hepatotoxicity Pulmonary fibrosis	Inhibits topoisomerase II from resealing double stranded breaks in DNA.
Irinotecan Camptosar®	Metastatic carcinoma of colon or rectum	Myelosuppression Anaphylaxis Pulmonary toxicity	Inhibits topoisomerase I from resealing single strand breaks in DNA
Teniposide Vumon®	Refractory childhood acute lymphoblastic leukemia	Severe myelosuppression Anaphylaxis	Inhibits topoisomerase II from resealing double stranded breaks in DNA.
Topotecan Hycamtin®	Metastatic carcinoma of the ovary, small cell lung cancer	Bone marrow suppression Neutropenia Interstitial lung disease	Same as above

Hematopoietic Drugs

Generic Name Brand Name	Clinical Use	Dose	Mechanism of Action
Epoetin Alpha Epogen®, Procrit®	Treats anemia	Adult, Cancer patient treated with chemotherapy: 150 units/kg SubQ 3 times a week or 40,000 units once weekly	Promotes the growth of red blood cells, erythropoiesis
Darbepoetin Aranesp®	Anemia	0.45 mcg/kg IV or SubQ weekly or 0.75 mcg/kg IV or SubQ every 2 weeks	Binds with erythropoietin receptors on erythrocyte progenitor cells.
Filgrastim (G-CSF) Neupogen®	Treats chemotherapy induced neutropenia	Children and adults IV or SubQ: 5 mcg/kg/day, use for upto 14 days or until ANC is 10,000/mm^3	Binds with receptors on progenitor cells causing their differentiation into neutrophils

Hematopoietic Drugs			
Generic Name Brand Name	Clinical Use	Dose	Mechanism of Action
Oprelvekin	Prevents severe throm-bocytopenia, thereby reducing the necessity of platelet transfusions	Adult, SubQ: 50 mcg/kg QD for 10-21 days, until post-nadir platelet count is 50,000 cells/ul or greater.	As a growth factor, oprelvekin stimulates the production of platelets.
Pegfilgrastim Neulasta®	Treats chemotherapy induced neutropenia	One single SubQ dose of 6mg per chemotherapy cycle. Do not ad-minister 14 days before or within 24 hours after the administration of cytotoxic chemotherapy.	Binds with receptors on progenitor cells causing their differentiation into neutrophils.
Sargramostim (GM-CSF) Leukine®	Treats chemotherapy induced neutropenia	Adult, AML, IV: 250 mcg/m^2/day, start about day 11 or 4 days follow-ing the completion of induction chemotherapy, if on day 10, bone marrow is less than 5% blasts.	Promotes the prolifer-ation of all blood cells, including white blood cells, eosinophils, mono-cytes and macrophages

Index

www.ingramcontent.com/pod-product-compliance
Lightning Source LLC
Chambersburg PA
CBHW051117200326
41518CB00016B/2533